Dedicated to my family
and to the memory of
my mother and father

Independent nursing practice with clients

Independent nursing practice with clients

M. Lucille Kinlein, R.N., B.A., M.S.N.E.
Independent Generalist Nurse
Visiting Professor,
University of Southern Mississippi

J. B. LIPPINCOTT COMPANY
PHILADELPHIA
New York   San Jose   Toronto

ISBN 0-397-54204-6
Library of Congress Catalog Card Number 77-3545
Printed in the United States of America
135798642

Library of Congress Cataloging in Publication Data

Kinlein, M. Lucille.
  Independent nursing practice with clients.

  Includes bibliographical references and index.
  1. Nursing—Philosophy. 2. Nursing—Practice.
I. Title. [DNLM: 1. Judgment. 2. Nursing.
3. Nursing care. 4. Nurse-patient relations.
5. Nurse practitioners. WY128 K55i]

RT84.5.K56   610.73′01

Contents

Introduction

In 1971, when I started my independent practice, I knew I would someday write about it. A rough draft was already taking shape in my mind as I sat in my office waiting for the first client. I knew that it would have to describe the frustration I had experienced as a professional nurse before setting up the practice, my search for the key to the problem, and the ultimate exit from the labyrinth of activities subsumed into an aggregate known—wrongly, I believe—as "medical care." In that maze, I could never identify a movement from "here" to "there" that I could call nursing. The "here" and "there" were always set by someone else, and I, the nurse, was always practicing between the two points. There was no nursing as an integrated whole, only the routine of performing isolated tasks, of doing things to, for, and with people—in relation to a *medical* problem.

I was professionally frustrated because I was attempting to implement what was syllogistically sound, but practically not possible; to reconcile the nursing classroom with the nursing practice setting; to end the beclouding of descriptions of nursing judgment, thought, or action by endless discussion and subtle twisting of meaning. I was frustrated by the semantic gyrations occurring during discussions of professional nursing. For example: "We should make professional judgments in nursing," nurses would agree. Then, however, each would add qualifications to that statement, and rationalizations weakening her stance. The discussion would then be dominated by sentences beginning, "But we shouldn't . . ." and, "We can't . . . ," until finally the nurses would arrive at a definition of judgment so distorted that it bore little resemblance to the real meaning of the word.

In this confusing way the contradictions were compounded and hence, what was defined as a nursing judgment between the hours of 11 P.M. and 7 A.M. was redefined as a medical judgment between the hours of 7 A.M. and 3 P.M. and as eclectic from 3 P.M. to 11 P.M.—the definitions being based on the timing of physicians' rounds in the hospital. Such mental gyrations have led to a continuing failure to appreciate and to discriminate among the real meanings of the words *health, illness, nursing* and *medicine*. "To nourish and sustain a person" cannot be identical with "to diagnose and treat an illness," nor can the episodic nature of medical care be identical with the continuing nature of helping one to stay healthy.

Nursing has been described as doing the obvious thing, or, again, as using common sense in a particular situation. But what is more complex than the obvious? And is not common sense the combination of a sound knowledge base with the tempering wisdom gained from experience, maintained in alignment with the immutability of nature? Because nursing is caring for a person, not caring for a thing, we have now to apply common sense to the most immutable feature—human nature—and so the complexity of the subjects disguises the obvious thing to be done, the obvious path to take and the obvious outcome to predicate. Is it not possible that a fresh light, a fresh perspective cast on the mutating fixtures of illness and disease—given by those caring for the persons with illness and disease—will change the nature of the fixtures? As Edmund Burke said, "They pity the plumage and forget the dying bird."

Or consider G. K. Chesterton's essay "On Lying in Bed," with its marvelous first sentence. "Lying in bed would be an altogether perfect and supreme experience if only one had a coloured pencil long enough to draw on the ceiling." He thinks it was only because Michelangelo was engaged in the activity of lying in bed that he realized how the roof of the Sistine Chapel might be made into an awesome imitation of the divine drama that could only be acted in the heavens. Chesterton goes on to say: "Misers get up early in the morning; and burglars, I am informed, get up the night before. It is the great peril of our society that all its mechanisms may grow more fixed while its spirit grows more fickle. A man's minor actions and arrangements ought to be free, flexible and creative, the things that should be unchangeable are his principles, his ideals. But with us the reverse is true; our views can change constantly; but our lunch does not change. Now, I should like men to have strong and rooted conceptions, but as for their lunch, let them have it sometimes in the garden, sometimes in bed, sometimes on the roof, sometimes in the top of a tree. Let them argue from the same first principles, but let them do it in a bed or a boat or a balloon."

It is the same great peril that plagues the profession of nursing. The professional nurse has allowed the mechanism to be fixed, the minor actions and arrangements to be unchanged. But during all these years the principles of nursing should have been fixed, and arguments should have been built on the premise of the unchanging concern of the nurse for care of the person—not on those things which are done for the person or to the person. In nursing, the fixed mechanisms have been the morning report, the bath, the temperature, pulse, and respiration, admission and discharge, preparation for the operating room, laboratory tests, medications, treatments, doctors' visits, etc. And we have maneuvered the person like an electronically guided missile into, around, over and alongside these unchanged minor arrangements, demanding change in the person to accommodate the charted pathway of nursing care in the traditional settings. Hence, we have a nursing approach to the colostomy patient, to the cardiac patient, to the diabetic patient and to the fracture patient. Perhaps the patient is duly programmed to fit the hospital or clinic routine because the nurse has been programmed to fit the needs of the institution and feels responsible for insuring the smooth coordination of the schedules and operation of the several departments of admissions, surgery, laboratory and X ray. Nursing has talked much about the need for change within the profession—change in the care of people—and then has changed forms and policies and rotation schedules, while nursing care goes on its way, furnishing grounds for jokes that constantly and clearly proclaim society's image of nursing and the professional nurse. Why do we lament the image and yet continue to assure its perpetuation by not changing nursing care? Are we afraid? Of what?

If the effectiveness of nursing is measured in terms of doing something, then, indeed, those traditional nursing activities assume importance in and of themselves. The criterion for measuring progress within the field of nursing could be whether or not the nurse knows the up-to-date changes in the technology spawning the techniques used in the care of the person. If one accepts that as a description of nursing in the professional sense, then one must accept the same definition of other professions, and ludicrous questions can be asked: How many patients did a physician see in a day? How many operations did a surgeon perform in a day? How many cases did a lawyer plead in a day? How many houses did an architect design in a day? How many paintings did an artist paint in a day? How many recitals did the violinist give in a day? If, however, more sensible criteria are used, then the evaluation of nursing effectiveness changes dramatically, and only the nurse can describe the progress a person makes as the result of the nurse's skills in giving care. Then the aimlessness of her action is eliminated and the practice of nursing is endowed with the unique quality of self-determination of the "here" and "there", of the starting point and the goal sought along the continuum of progress.

And that is why I went into independent practice, offering to the people who would seek my services these features: availability, accessibility, accuracy, accountability and autonomy. I offered the skills of one nurse to one person at a time, and this person I called a "client."* In addition, I set up five criteria for myself in my practice: I would practice in a setting in which I would be the only professional rendering care; I would subsidize my own practice; I would charge a fee for my services; I would practice as a generalist; I would give care

* See explanation of "client" on page 8

within an articulated concept of nursing care, and I would validate it as far as possible to the level of theory. *This final criterion was the most important one because it was imperative that I be able to articulate the difference between what I was doing and what doctors were doing before I hung out my shingle.* The most widely held concept of nursing at that time was (and I believe still is) that nursing is the extension of medicine; the nurse is the extension of the physician practicing medical care. I have the concept, however, that nursing is properly the extension of the client. I see nursing as an entity in itself among the professions in the health field; I see it as a profession in which the professional nurse will appropriately set the direction of nursing by including para-nursing or nonprofessional nursing groups when planning a system of nursing care for the person who needs nursing that requires various levels of preparation.

When I first considered writing about my practice, I thought of the field of nursing education. Because for twenty-four years I had been primarily an educator, my thoughts naturally turned to the academic preparation for the profession of nursing. One day when I was in my office following an appointment with a client, it occurred to me that I would have to write about how my practice might affect the curriculum in schools of nursing. For the first time in nursing history, I was gathering data in the purest form possible. In the past, research had been done on nursing practice when a *medical* need brought the person into contact with the nurse. The study of nursing under conditions with multiple variables in the form of therapies, personnel and sundry environmental factors yields conclusions of questionable value. But in my practice I had reduced the factors to two: client and nurse. I had eliminated all the uncontrollable variables.

The person crossing the threshold of my office came for a reason of his own—the visit was not an adjunct to a previously established therapeutic regimen—and what he told me I put into a pattern of thought consistent with the articulated concept of nursing that I knew I had to have before hanging out my shingle. Thus, analyzing client histories would give to nursing the first classifications of nursing determinations under the conditions just described. The analysis of the nursing measures I had taken in light of the client's expressed need would give to the nursing world the first detailed documentation of nursing judgment and nursing action, and of their results within a formulated concept. Of such data is the structured body of knowledge in a practice discipline constructed. From such data hypotheses can be made for graduate study, while baccalaureate students can study the state of the art at a particular time in its development.

Perhaps I have sacrificed depth in favor of breadth in selecting the thrust of this book, but among the thousands of questions asked of me over the last four years, this question predominates: What is your independent nursing practice all about? I have attempted to answer in part some of the angles incorporated in this question. My independent nursing practice is all about one professional nurse taking seriously the meaning of the words *professional, judgment, decision, authority, responsibility, accountability, truth, justice,* and *charity.* It is about one professional nurse who, after making a commitment and devising a way to meet that commitment, helps people who come to her for help. Finally, it is about one professional nurse helping other nurses to fructify their multiple talents to help many other people. This book presents the rationale for independent practice, for giving care, for putting nursing in its proper place in the health field as a practice discipline that is the extension of the person, the client.

One final, personal observation I feel it only fair to make about the frame of reference within which my own theory and practice of nursing exists. I live and work as a practicing Roman Catholic. Professionally, personally and intellectually, this has consequences: to take two very obvious examples, I do not accept abortion and euthanasia; in nursing, as in medical practice, I recognize the existence of many other problems with moral dimensions. That might be called a negative consequence. Positively, and much more important, my religious convictions mean, among other things touching my profession, that I reverence the human body and that I recognize the inestimable dignity of every human person. While bending every professional effort to alleviate pain and suffering and to prolong life, I recognize and accept the mysterious ways in which Providence manifests itself in every human life, even when this involves pain, suffering and untimely death.

With Teilhard de Chardin, in *The Divine Milieu*—one of the best treatments I know of the spiritual aspects of the intellectual/professional life—I believe that "God truly waits for us in all things, unless indeed He advances to meet us [but] the manifestation of His divine presence in no way disturbs the harmony of our human [read *professional*] attitude, but on the contrary brings it its true form and perfection."

Acknowledgments

The author wishes to express her deepest appreciation and thanks to the following persons and groups of persons who—often without their knowing it—have been of inestimable help in bringing this book into being.

To all of the clients who have come to me since June, 1971, whose faith in my nursing theories and abilities helped me so much to maintain confidence in the validity of my concepts and their implementation. Special mention must be made of Mrs. Albertina Haynes, who became my client in 1972. At that time, at 75 years of age, she pursued this course of action: she went to four physicians in separate locations and asked them if they would proceed with her medical care using the results of the laboratory tests done when she came to me for nursing care. Three replied in the negative and the physician who finally agreed has his office quite some distance from her home. As of this day she still goes to see him as a matter of principle, even though she is now 80 years old.

To Miss Dorothea Orem, R.N., Scholar of Nursing, whose basic theory of the self-care agency approach to nursing was my original inspiration, and to the members of the Nursing Development Conference Group, of which Miss Orem was one of the prime movers. From them, as one of the members, I gained many invaluable insights into nursing theory and its applications. I wish to stress most emphatically that many of the ways in which I have utilized what I learned from Miss Orem and the Group are of my own devising; and I trust that my modifications of the concept will not be interpreted as a violation of the integrity of the original concept.

To Mrs. Patti Alberger, expert in editorial matters, "manuscript doctor" and professional journalist, for her help in the articulation of a new concept in nursing through a book which is partly an autobiographical account, partly the presentation of a concept, and partly a textbook of professional nursing care. Her expertise has enabled me to send off to the publisher a coherent, cohesive presentation of an idea put into practice.

To Mrs. Karin Thompson, professional nurse and executive secretary. She came to me when I needed her most, as one of the many blessings vouchsafed to me since I began my independent practice of nursing.

To Mrs. Roxanne Stigers, Administrator of Collingswood Nursing Center, whose professional support and friendship have been enduring.

To Miss Nellie Lee Powell, Librarian of the School of Nursing at the Catholic University of America, who has for many years put her talents and her friendship—and often her very house—at my disposal.

To Mrs. Barbara Bauer, who gives me a room in her house as my office in Green Bay, Wisconsin.

And finally to all professional colleagues and friends—and I am fortunate that in so many cases the terms are synonymous—whose support has been invaluable.

M. L. K.

chapter one

View of nursing past and a vision for the future

Through the years the nursing profession has evolved largely in concert with the medical profession to which it has been a handmaiden. However, the nursing profession by itself *has* shown some signs of change. Until very recently, most nurses were trained in three-year programs at schools of nursing associated with hospitals. There is no question that excellent nurses were graduated from most of these schools. However, academically speaking, they were graduates of curricula for which there was no equivalent—hence no recognition of value—in the educational system of the United States. They were terminal programs and did not serve as a basis for continuing education within the accepted levels of higher education. The reason was that, in the hospital curriculum, the content of liberal arts and science courses had been mutilated and narrowed in the interest of meeting the criterion of relevance to nursing. There were, for example, chemistry *for nurses*, psychology *for nurses*, and so on. When drafting the syllabus for such a course, many faculty members used a verbal scissors when they asked: What are the implications of this subject matter for nursing? In their view, those implications had to be nailed down before material from the sciences and the humanities could be included in the curriculum. Two glaring errors in this approach

1

were not picked up by well-intentioned educators. The first was the assumption that a definition of nursing in fact exists—a definition that is universally accepted and that is upheld, albeit tacitly, by all members of the profession. The second was the practice of selecting content from whole bodies of knowledge with an eye to immediate, restricted purpose—a selection that staked out the boundaries of nursing action and thus diminished creativity.

Thus, graduates of these nursing programs emerged competent in giving injections, administering backrubs, taking temperatures, teaching patients, reassuring patients, and performing a number of other tasks associated with the medical needs of patients. During the doctor shortage brought on by World War II, nurses often substituted for physicians in performing the primary medical actions of diagnosis and initiation of treatment.

After the war, there was a murmur of change in nursing, evidenced by the movement toward more extensive educational preparation for nurses. Baccalaureate degree programs in nursing were offered. However, the same glaring errors persisted throughout this phase. Graduates of three-year nursing schools about to enter college would say, "We all know about nursing, so why do we have to take nursing courses?" And faculty members would say, "They have had their nursing major, so in order to meet the degree requirement they need only complete the first and second year courses in general college subjects." The less than sage advice given to high school students by parents and counselors was: "Get your nursing courses first in a three-year program; you can always go back to get your college degree." Acquiring at a later date the foundation on which the study of nursing should have been built was interpreted as progress. Such academic foolishness merited the put-down by nurses of collegiate programs in nursing as inferior to hospital programs in nursing content. Educators in other fields had difficulty reconciling the sequence of nursing major first, foundation later—and with good reason.

The same errors were being perpetrated and perpetuated. Leaders in nursing still assumed that there was a universal definition of nursing to which every nurse subscribed, and they structured learning and teaching accordingly. When the murmur of change in nursing grew louder in the 1950s, therefore, it was inevitable that the direction would remain the same as before. The pressure on nurses to get master's degrees in nursing to qualify them for teaching, supervision and administration paralleled the granting of federal funds for this purpose. The lamentable aspect of this situation was that, in essence, the nursing content had not changed from that of the three-year hospital program.

The knowledge explosion in the 1960s in all branches of learning, but particularly in physiology, biochemistry and bioengineering, gave rise to new and increasingly complex medical technologies. Doctors needed help, and nurses were taught how to help them. As a result, the nurse specialist was born—the heart-lung nurse, the critical care nurse, the trauma unit nurse, the coronary care nurse, the ostomy nurse, the dialysis nurse and so on. The nursing literature called this emergence a change in nursing. I submit that change had indeed occurred, but that it was not in nursing. It was in medical technology, and nurses were taught how to make decisions about a person's medical condition based on data gathered by means of the new technology. Such close working relationships with physicians did have a noteworthy outcome. There was an awakening on the part of many physicians to the intellectual capacity of nurses. The simultaneous emergence of medicine by machine as a result of technological advances meant, however, that these thinking nurses became enmeshed in tasks of growing complexity that could have been performed just as easily by well-trained technicians. Consequently, personal contact with the patient was abdicated and was delegated to nonprofessional personnel trained not in general patient care, but in the performance of specific tasks. Or, in some settings, nurses became the guardians of bureaucracy, their hours consumed with paperwork and red tape instead of with nursing care given directly to people. To the person at the receiving end of these activities— the patient—the human touch supposedly provided by nurses must have seemed distant.

At the same time, the person in the hospital bed was gaining an awareness of health and medicine unparalleled in history. In the past, matters of health were not spoken of so candidly as they are now. The atmosphere of mystery concerning medicine is declining, as more and more lay persons demand more knowledge about their bodies and minds and a larger role in their care and maintenance. The physician is no longer left unchallenged by the recipients of his care, as more of his patients assume the right to examine what the doctor ordered and why. The lay person has been educated through various media and citizen groups; he is amassing knowledge; and he wants to use that knowledge to stay healthy.

There is a definite change, then, in the health expectations of the lay person. These expectations are causing him to demand health services beyond the ones traditionally available. For example, before World War II, this sequence of events dominated the thinking of the layman: I am well—I get sick—I go to the doctor—I may go to the hospital. I get nursing care when I am in the hospital—and I might get nursing care after I return home—when I get better I will not get nursing care—but I will continue with medical care, at least for a while. The new thinking, however, follows this progression: I am well—I want to stay that way—I am aware that there are reasons for needing help in addition to the medical care that is given after an illness has been diagnosed and treated—there is a time when, although my medical needs have been met by a physician, my other needs have not been met, and I need the services of other professional persons in the health field.

What is needed, precisely, is the professional nurse—a nurse practicing in a way that has not yet been encountered in the health care system. People are recognizing that they need nursing assistance and perhaps other kinds of assistance to stay healthy; nursing and other kinds of assistance when they are ill and under medical therapy; and nursing and other kinds of assistance following an episode of illness. A "new" nurse is needed in all phases of the health-illness continuum. That new nurse—educated in a system in which the glaring errors have been corrected—will be identified by the way in which she uses her unlimited and ever-growing knowledge base and by the goal that she pursues in giving nursing care to the person seeking her help. (The goal will be distinct from a medical goal.) To understand fully how radical this seemingly simple thought is, it is necessary to discuss the "old" way and the "old" goals.

In the practice setting, the nurse's knowledge was applied mainly to the effective execution of the medical plan of care. Her decisions were based on the scientific principles underlying the therapeutic measures that had been instituted for a particular condition for which the patient had sought medical advice. The degree of complexity of the judgments made by the nurse many times depended upon the degree to which she could act without transgressing the boundary of medical practice. Clearly, the attainment of medical goals can be seen as the nurse's goal when she carries out such instructions from the physician as, "Don't tell the patient he has cancer." "Don't tell the patient he is dying." "Don't tell the patient what his temperature or blood pressure is." Yet the nursing textbooks teach that the nurse should "reassure" the patient in moments of stress and encourage him to talk about his fears. The nurse's frustration because of this contradiction has been intense. The fusion and confusion of nursing and medicine have reinforced the untenable position in which the nurse has been placed in not being able to carry out measures which in her judgment would benefit the patient.

Nursing education has, for the most part, aided in perpetuating this untenable position. The knowledge that a nurse acquired through traditional programs was oriented toward pathology, disease, medical treatments and pharmacology. In the classroom, injunctions to use this knowledge about the patient's signs and symptoms, or his medications, or his prognosis, were accompanied by enjoinders to refrain from disclosing information that the doctor did not want the person to have (again in contradiction of the alleged nursing mission of reducing patient anxiety). Many times the nurse knew the patient as a person much better than the physician did. Furthermore, the decisions made by the nurse in regard to the patient's medical condition were required to be extremely accurate so that the physician could evaluate changes and revise therapy accordingly. Surely, this is an example of contradiction, in view of the limited communication permitted between patient and nurse, as a matter of policy.

Thus nursing education has fostered a distressing dichotomy in the nurse's perception of her role. Educators insisted that the nurse keep abreast of the latest changes in drugs, treatments and pathology, but never changed the core of the curriculum—which should have been nursing. This absence of nursing content from the curriculum accounts for the hours upon hours and effort upon effort invested by so many nurses in meetings called to plan change—all fruitless in the long run, because nursing had not been defined. In both nursing practice and education, then, the "mechanisms" and "minor arrangements" described by Chesterton received attention while nursing went undefined, the victim of an apparent fickleness of the intellect that nurtured such beliefs as "Everybody knows what nursing is—why define it? Stop wasting time and get on with it!"

The missing link in the identification of this "nursing" that everyone supposedly recognizes has been a conceptual framework within which nursing could be practiced and recorded—a framework that could be taught along with the structured body of nursing knowledge. If a conceptual framework were defined, it would have to be observable in practice settings. The rockbound, steeped-in-tradition settings of nursing in the past have not been amenable to changes that would have permitted observation of the concept in action. In addition, the needs of people traditionally classified as "nursing needs" were actually needs that had been identified as a result of some medical condition. They were called nursing needs because nurses met those needs. One need not ponder long to realize that, without criteria to identify a need as being within the field of nursing, there were no limits on what might be called nursing, as long as the nurse had the capacity, willingness—and unquestioning attitude—to do whatever she was told was her responsibility. The proffered rationale by nurses and others that the patient would ultimately benefit if the nurse helped the doctor, or sorted laundry, or gave out medications, or filled out forms and reports, or answered the telephone is, at best, a limp excuse for not wanting to be bothered with definitions.

One *must* be concerned with the definition of nursing needs. A graphic presentation of nursing in the medical framework and of nursing in a framework of its own can be useful in arriving at a definition.

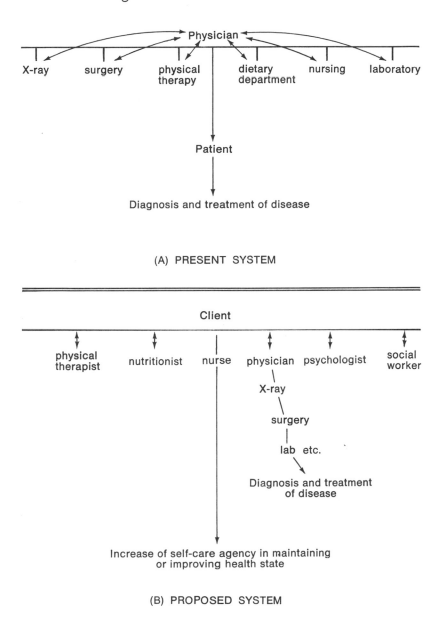

Figure 1–1   (A) Present System. (B) Proposed System.

As Figure 1–A shows, nursing in the present medical framework is an extension of medicine—the nurse assisting the physician in his goal of diagnosing and treating illness. The present system isolates the patient and the physician in the only legitimate relationship. Members of the other fields have contact with the patient only through the physician, and usually the information given consists only of data that will answer the physician's specific questions regarding a possible pathological condition. Consequently, the patient has access to information about his body only as it relates to a possible disease. He is thus denied broader knowledge about his health state that he could use in maintaining and in adopting a self-care regimen. Nursing in the medical framework is but one of many services used by the physician in the medical treatment of his patient.

In Figure 1–B, the person—referred to as the client*—holds a different position. The nurse is in direct primary contact with the client if he feels he needs a nurse. The nurse is an extension of the client, not of the physician, and the nurse/client relationship is formed around the goal of increasing the self-care agency of the client in maintaining and improving his health state. The client in this system can explore the full gamut of his health state and can reconcile his goals and life patterns with that health state. He makes decisions about his needs and is free to call on the appropriate resource people in the health field. In this system, medicine—the diagnosing and treating of disease—is part of a total health system. If it is desired, the

---

* I refer to persons who come to me as "clients," not as "patients." In using the term "client" I feel I am free of the restrictive connotation of illness that is intrinsic to the word "patient." Use of the word "patient" puts nursing in a sequential position, as in the traditional settings; whereas the nursing that I practice is in a position of initiation, of independence. In addition, I think it is important for nurses to establish legitimate relationships with the persons for whom they are caring, so that the important feature of accountability can be observed. The word "client" seems to convey this legitimate relationship of the nurse in primary contact with her client. Also, the word "patient" in the traditional medical system connotes passiveness: the patient is diagnosed, treated, given prescriptions and orders regarding therapy. The word "client" does not have this passive connotation. In the nursing relationship, the client is active: he seeks the help of the nurse, and part of the nursing care that is given is helping the client to recognize and communicate his needs. The client must, in my concept of nursing, be active. He asks questions and receives full answers; he takes an active part as we assess his self-care agency and as we initiate improvements. Thus, the word "client" seems to be appropriate in conveying many important aspects of my nursing practice.

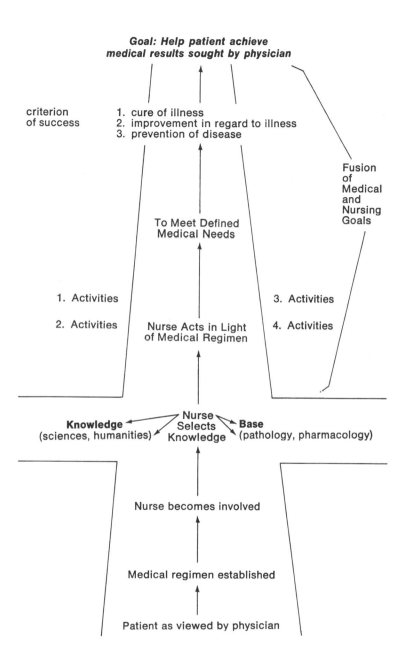

Goal: **Help patient achieve
medical results sought by physician**

criterion
of success

1. cure of illness
2. improvement in regard to illness
3. prevention of disease

Fusion
of
Medical
and
Nursing
Goals

To Meet Defined
Medical Needs

1. Activities

2. Activities

Nurse Acts in Light
of Medical Regimen

3. Activities

4. Activities

Knowledge
(sciences, humanities)

Nurse
Selects
Knowledge

Base
(pathology, pharmacology)

Nurse becomes involved

Medical regimen established

Patient as viewed by physician

Figure 1–2   Sequence of Nursing in a Medical Model

nurse, as an extension of the client, can collate the information gathered by other professionals and help him to apply that broad knowledge to a self-care regimen. Nursing in this system is not one of the many services used in treating disease, but one of the many professional services available for maintaining health.

Let us now take a closer look at nursing in both the present and proposed systems:

Figure 1–2 illustrates nursing as it exists in the present medical system. The person's medical needs as defined by the physician direct the actions of the nurse. The criterion of success—the prevention of, cure of or improvement in a diseased condition—encapsulates for the nurse the reason for unidirectional action based on her study and knowledge of disease, of pathology—of what is amiss in a person. The nurse is an extension of the physician, assisting him in the performance of medical tasks. In this framework, the nurse often unconsciously makes the person an adjunct to the goal to be achieved —the means to an end. The phenomenon occurs as a result of the burden, pressure and responsibility of gathering accurate medical data so that effective medical therapy can be accomplished. Hence, precisely what nursing is in this situation is obscured. Because she is engrossed in her medical tasks, the nurse may not recognize needs or, if she discerns them, may not have the time to engage in nursing in light of those needs. The medical framework does not permit the establishment of a legitimate nurse/client relationship (one not directly related to the medical condition in question) within which the nurse can help the person to recognize and communicate needs related to his health state and can work together with him toward improvement in his self-care agency. It has been an irony of our system that a person must usually be ill in order to see a nurse, who could, potentially, provide all-encompassing services related to his health state. When he does see a nurse, she has entered the picture only after a medical regimen has been established, and her actions are limited in view of that regimen. Thus, the nursing potential remains unfulfilled.

Figure 1–3 shows how nursing could function outside the medical model. In the nursing model there is, first of all, the establishment of a legitimate nurse/client rela-

Sequence of Nursing in a Nursing Model
As Contrasted with Nursing in a
Medical Model

Point of Departure: The Person Asks for Nursing Care by a Specific Nurse
and a Legitimate Relationship is Established When the
Nurse Accepts the Responsibility, a Fee is Established,
and the Person Becomes the Nurse's Client.

This professional relationship marks the beginning of a definite but extremely delicate interaction which has as its hallmark a dynamic flow between two individuals. No other health professional contact maintains so constant a focus on the person even when a painful physical condition is being explored, a psychological condition is being explored, or a decision-making process is underway. There is a fluidity that characterizes the nursing interaction, a flow, a continuously dynamic state. Such motion demands that the client be uppermost in the focus of the nurse—not the physical pain or the psychological state or the decision being made. In other words, time must be given for physical pain to be handled, for psychological pain to be expressed, for helplessness to be admitted. At a given moment, the measure selected by the nurse as most helpful to the client might be the expression of factual knowledge found in the scientific literature—the words themselves lifting the burden of the body and the mind from the self of the person. The decision by the nurse to use certain information and to tell it to the person in a certain manner is a nursing judgment, because the goal is to help the person with his need at that particular moment. So, the more knowledge the nurse has, the more opportunities are open to her to select appropriate verbal vehicles to help the person in his self-care. There is a kind of tailoring effect that must be carried out in the acts of nursing, and the skill of the nurse is challenged when she deals with the tailoring process, from two aspects: (1) the vast body of scientific knowledge and (2) the uniqueness of each individual in regard to his stated need. The pieces selected from (1) and from (2) must be as perfect a match as possible. Thus, in a sense, nursing care in any given period of time—minutes or hours—produces the following sequence:

Change is caused in the person through
use of individual measures . . .

which cause a change in the person, . . .

thus demanding another decision on the part of
the nurse to

cause further change in the person through
use of individualized measures. . . .

And so the process continues in the presence of the person about whom the nurse is making judgments; it continues in the presence of the person for, whom the nurse might be rendering physical care—at which time the act of TOUCH assumes measurable and immeasurable effects.

In summary,

The client asks for nursing care ⟶ The nurse in her judgment
focuses on the
uniqueness of

This individual,
this person, in his ⟵
stated need.

The client is changed,
however subtly, and   continues to ask
for nursing care ⟶ The nurse
continues to make
judgments based on
the uniqueness of

This individual. ⟵

In nursing, the challenge is in the focus of the person as the formal object. The pitfall is in the generalizing about the individual in light of the specifics of the condition in which he presents himself in need to the nurse.

Figure 1–3 Sequence of Nursing in a Nursing Model

tionship. There is no predetermined result, such as the diagnosis of illness, to restrict the nurse in the direction she may take in response to the client's expressed needs. Nursing occurs from the outset, as the nurse helps the client to recognize and communicate those needs and to view them in the light of his health state and goals. During all phases, there is free-flowing interaction with the client. Thus, new needs continue to surface as the nursing process continues. This continuous recognition can take place because the nurse's vision is not narrowed by a specific medical target; it is all-encompassing, since it takes into account the client's broader health picture.

From these illustrations, it is obvious that nurses are confronted with a choice of direction, as Figure 1–4 shows. The right to choose either path of practice is, of course, the nurse's prerogative. However, if she chooses to practice in the medical framework, if she chooses to be an extension of the physician, she incurs the burden of explaining, as nursing, the results of her practice. This statement is not intended as a put-down of nurses' worth in the medical system. However, the work of these practitioners can be correctly labeled with a number of other terms, because traditionally so many diverse activities have been called "nursing" that the word itself has lost its meaning. I am attempting to put a meaning into the word, and suggesting that other functions be named more precisely, according to what is actually being done.

Inherent in the new nursing framework that I am suggesting are several important notions of nursing which must be postulated and followed. They will emerge for further elaboration in subsequent chapters:

1. A professional nurse must be known by the care she gives to the person, not by the care she gives to the physician, to the X-ray department or to the laboratory staff, etc.

2. Knowledge is a necessity, and this knowledge should be used in meeting the needs of the persons she is caring for, not in making a medical diagnosis or in initiating therapy, which are the two functions that identify the practice of medicine.

3. The more it is obviously necessary to do something medically for a person, the less need there is for a professional

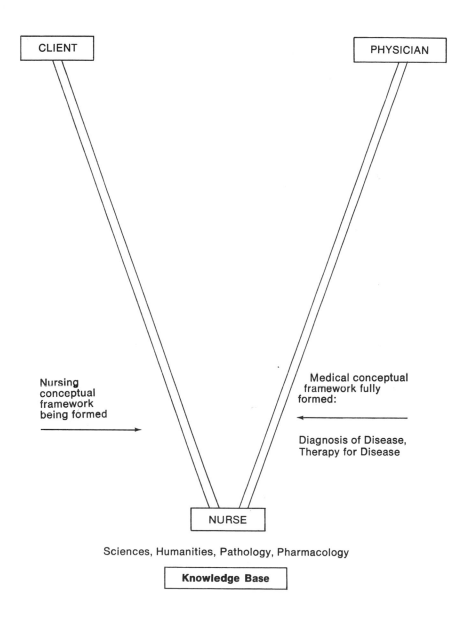

Figure 1–4 Choice of Direction Confronting the Nurse

nursing judgment about that "something" that is required. If the degree of necessity diminishes, then medical judgment is still needed, because that is the art of the practice of medicine.

4. The professional nurse must accept and incorporate into her concept of professional practice the crystallization and articulation of a theory of nursing that will enable her to be absolutely sure that she is practicing nursing, and that will guide her safely through those gray areas of overlap of nursing with related disciplines that will always be there. Without a theory of nursing, we will never be able to structure a body of knowledge from the excellent nursing care that has been given through the years.

5. We do not know the professional nursing needs of the client simply because we know the medical needs of the patient.

6. It takes time to give professional nursing care to a client; if there is not sufficient time to assess a client's nursing need, then no professional nursing care can be given. We cannot implement that which we have not assessed. An activity can be done to, for, or with a person, but this is not in and of itself nursing, even if a nurse does it.

7. A professional nurse is an extension of the client, not an extension of the physician.

8. A professional nurse should be and can be independent in any setting.

9. Activities do not define a professional's practice.

Growing out of the new framework and notions, of course, is the most dramatic new application of nursing —the independent practice. For in nursing as distinct from medicine (as has been seen in the illustrations), the various needs of the person are viewed in relation to the professional person best able to fill those needs. Thus, the person seeks nursing care in a setting not necessarily associated with the practice of medicine. With the change in the layman's health expectations and knowledge, it may be assumed that this seeking out will occur. Indeed, it *is* occurring today. Chapter 3 will explain how. But first, Chapter 2 will articulate the conceptual foundation upon which this new nursing structure must be built.

chapter two

Conceptual
foundation needed
to initiate change:
self-care concept

The self-care concept in health recognizes and emphasizes the inherent human attribute of individual domain over one's actions. From the time I began to study the concept, I sensed that its application would give the nursing profession greater freedom in providing health care to people. The nursing literature contained fragments of other conceptual approaches to the practice of nursing, but in my view they were inadequate in terms of the nurse's control over nursing care. Patient advocacy as a concept did not and does not convey the essence of a nursing concept to me. The notion of acting in behalf of someone, acting for someone's welfare, similarly fails. The main reason for this failure lies in the detachment of the nurse from the person being helped. Furthermore, the notion invites a flirtation with the peril of passivity on the part of the one being helped. At the other extreme of interpreting dependence and independence as it relates to the involvement of the person being helped, it should be noted that self-care does not mean letting the person "do things for himself" in a system devised by the nurse.

I can trace my development of a concept by showing the mental constructs with which I functioned at various stages of my career—stages leading to the development of

15

the self-care concept and its refinement, as I applied it in my independent practice.

During the 1950s and early 1960s, when I was teaching in the baccalaureate program, and as my medical knowledge grew, I would approach patients with this mental construct:

Contact with Patient	*Continuous thinking during Contact*	
My knowledge of pathology, signs and symptoms, pharmacology, probable treatment.	Be careful; don't make a diagnosis; don't suggest that the therapy is not particularly appropriate; cut the line as fine as possible; don't miss anything; if a subtle sign or symptom is missed, it could mean complication or even death.	What am I going to do with the information that this patient is giving me? I've listened to her; she cooperates well and responds well to all of her treatments and medications; I've checked and have refrained from giving the impression that either all is well or that all is not well.

When I was teaching cardiovascular nursing at the master's level, I experienced an even greater degree of frustration than I had known at the baccalaureate level. I knew I was perpetuating the shortcomings of nursing, compounding the problem, and in desperation I figured out that the answer might lie in placing emphasis on the physiological aspects of the cardiovascular system—on the normal. But where did that leave the medications, the treatments and the disease? Whither would this approach lead? My mental construct was this:

Contact with Patient	*Continuous Thinking During Contact*	
Increased (and constantly increasing) knowledge of pathology, signs and symptoms, pharmacology, probable treatment.	If I use this knowledge, how will I identify the results of its use as nursing? Result: reluctance to use this knowledge at all. I began to shrink from the clinical areas—the hub of technological activity.	I recognized that the person had a right to know what I knew; but without a concept of nursing I would be using the knowledge for a medical goal. Hence, I retreated from the patients and sought refuge in the study of physiology and in my search for a concept of nursing.

In order to break away from this restrictive mode of thought, yet still use all of my knowledge, I reasoned thus: Nursing is different from any other profession in the health field because the nurse directs her actions in nursing in a way that differs in nature and degree from the way in which members of other professions in the health field direct theirs. The closeness of contact, the continuous and extremely personal features of the relationship between the nurse and the other person are without parallel in the care given by other health professionals. Indeed, in the traditional settings this fact was observed and often given as a reason—albeit an invalid one—for the nurse to assume unwarranted responsibilities, to do things that, organizationally speaking, were in the purview of other departments during the week (but not on the weekends, because the departments were closed); during the day (but not during the evening and night hours). So, based on what the nursing literature said about the continuously personal element that was unequalled outside of nursing, and based on what I felt had characterized nursing care in the traditional settings, I would present to the person seeking my services the therapeutic elements and qualities that I possess.

I took the self-care concept in nursing and applied it to an individual's health state—as opposed to an individual's medical state. In so doing, I was tackling the biggest unknown of all, namely, health. Because lay persons had been taught about health only from the viewpoint of how sick they were not, or of what illness they could keep from getting, and because research is geared to and funded for the identification of aspects of diagnosis and treatment of disease, the literature is lacking in guidelines for the scientific identification of health states. Indeed, when health is discussed, it is largely in terms of the protection of the individual against some illness to which his particular population is prone.

The nursing approach I chose to take can be described further by examining the spectrum of health and illness and the positions that the professions of nursing and medicine respectively take in regard to the entire continuum. Both professions are interested in the entire continuum, of course, but the approach from *health* is completely different from the approach from *illness*. The following figure, a health continuum, serves to illustrate the two perspectives:

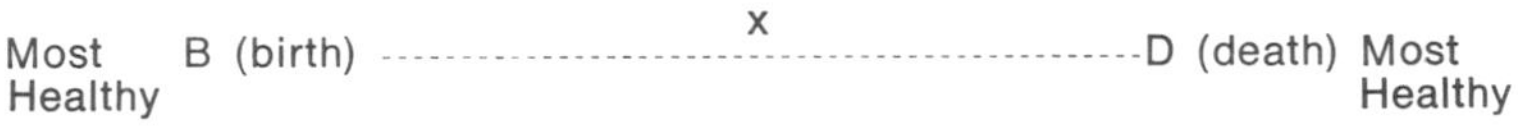

<pre>
                                        x
Most   B (birth) --D (death) Most
Healthy   Healthy
</pre>

Figure 2–1

Inasmuch as a criterion of absolute health is unattainable, health as a state must be considered in a relative sense. Let us assume that the majority of people have an extended, as opposed to a shortened, span of life prior to death, and that there are varying degrees of acute illness anywhere along the continuum. In Figure 2–1, B represents the best possible state of health at a given time and D the worst possible state of health at a given time. In general, medicine views medical effectiveness from the starting point of D. The person did not die; therefore medicine was effective. Moreover, unconsciousness is not as bad as death, consciousness is not as bad as unconsciousness, limited mobility is not as bad as paralysis, having only one leg is not as bad as having no legs—so that by the time midpoint x is reached, the medical appraisal might be a favorable one, as Figure 2–2 shows.

Nursing, on the other hand, should view nursing effectiveness from the starting point of B, generally the healthiest condition an individual can be in. Maintaining that health state should be the goal of nursing and a measure of its effectiveness. As the features of the healthy state diminish, the person becomes less healthy, and as the person moves through

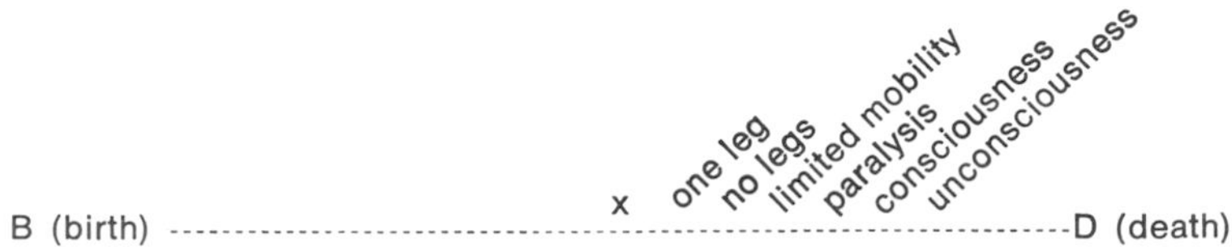

Health Continuum, Medical Appraisal

Figure 2–2

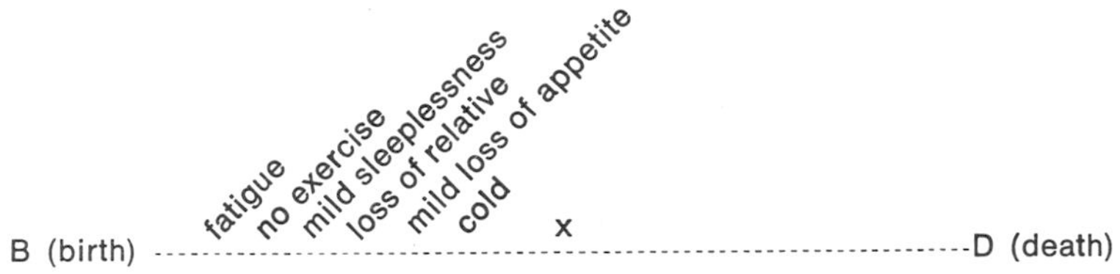

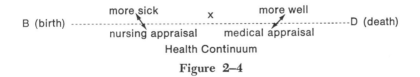

Health Continuum, Nursing Appraisal

Figure 2–3

time under conditions that reduce his maximum health state but
do not render him ill, as he reaches midpoint *x*, the nursing appraisal is an unfavorable one, as shown in Figure 2–3.

The fusion of the two viewpoints at midpoint
x results in two conflicting positions concerning how healthy a
person is, as seen in Figure 2–4. To the nurse, he is *more sick*
than well, and to the physician he is *more well* than sick. The
fact that there is such a dearth of research on the positive health
state is evidence that health standards in the United States have
been based largely on the progression from the worst to the
better state, and on the desire to prevent the most incapacitating
illness from occurring.

B (birth) ---------------------more sick-------x------more well----------------D (death)
                          nursing appraisal   medical appraisal
                              Health Continuum

Figure 2–4

Much of the time, of course, the perspective of the health professional will be reflected in the approach that he takes with
respect to the care of a given individual.

The focus of the nurse on the *health* state of
the individual is at once more difficult and more important because of the one big question in the field of health which has
not been satisfactorily answered: Why are healthy people
healthy? Surely, an individual's daily personal care habits must
play a large part in the determination of whether health can be
retained or regained. The self-care practices of individuals must

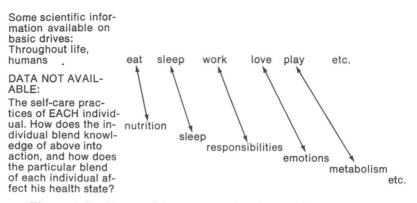

Some scientific infor-
mation available on
basic drives:
Throughout life,
humans .

DATA NOT AVAIL-
ABLE:
The self-care prac-
tices of EACH individ-
ual. How does the in-
dividual blend knowl-
edge of above into
action, and how does
the particular blend
of each individual af-
fect his health state?

eat   sleep   work   love   play   etc.

nutrition

sleep

responsibilities

emotions

metabolism

etc.

Figure 2–5   Universal Actions Translated into Individual Actions

in fact be a pivotal point, and hence should be focused on as a source of information for valid nursing data and medical data. But individuals lack knowledge about those self-care practices that would benefit their health states. This absence of information can be seen in Figure 2–5.

QUESTION:

1.   To what extent do the pluses and minuses of an individual's self-care practices affect his health state, which is also unknown?

2.   If information about the self-care practices of *many* individuals were gathered when they are healthy, would these facts lead us to a more effective way of handling any deviation from the health state when and if it occurs?

The concept of self-care health practices which constitutes the nursing framework within which I would give care in my practice would be applied thus:

Contact with Client	*Continuous thinking during Contact*	
Person would state the reason he came to see me . . . he would talk about his care of him- self.	This data would pro- vide the pivot on which my nursing care would turn . . . and a change in self-care practices should take place . . . which would feed into an identification of . . .	Body of scientific data about self-care practices and their effectiveness.

The preceding material supports and justifies the position that nursing is a profession distinctly different from the profession of medicine. Indeed, the episodic nature of *illness* in the health continuum, contrasted with the ongoing nature of *health*, plays havoc with the traditional concept of being under a doctor's care after a limited period of contact with the doctor—a situation resembling the somewhat unavailing circumstance of being cared for by remote control. Care by a physician is needed intermittently, sporadically, throughout life. The physician gets to look at the individual's health continuum mainly on those isolated occasions when symptoms of illness appear. In keeping with the concept of self-care practices, care by a nurse is needed on a more continuing basis. The nurse views the health continuum of an individual in its entirety, and when and if illness occurs, she views that illness in the context of the individual's total health picture as she, through her nursing care, has learned to know it. Thus nursing, because of its quality of continuity, which is the essence of nursing care—assumes an umbrella-like form that encompasses the other health professions.

A caveat is in order. The apparent simplicity of the concept as expressed in words that seem so clear constitutes a hazard to a professional nurse, who might read *about* the concept and confuse that acquaintance with *knowledge* of the concept. The temptation to feel secure in practicing nursing according to the concept might be quite strong. But a concept of nursing needs to be studied and analyzed before it is applied. The importance of judgment as an element of the concept of self-care cannot be overstressed. The contrast between performing according to what the nurse learned as nursing and practicing according to a concept of nursing can be perceived in the nature of the action. In the traditional setting, nursing care carries with it the element of certainty; i.e., the reason that a nurse engages in a nursing action is known before the contact with the patient is made. There is a scientific, validated reason for the medicine to be carried into the patient's room, for the treatment to be administered, for the vital signs to be monitored. In other words, the need of the person is identified *before* the nurse gives care. And the precise care given is usually the result of an order given by another professional, a physician. In such cases, the *judgment* the nurse exercises is relatively minimal.

So when a *new* technique is learned, it is wrapped around the old concept, and confusion about "new nursing" results. Similarly, if a nurse has not changed her basic concept of nursing, she will wrap the new words around the old concept, and ultimately be dismayed at the ineffectiveness of the "new concept."

In my own practice, as I translated the concept into action, I found myself stressing the positive aspect of health and freeing myself of the medical constraints of the negative approach to health. My concept at this time can be shown in this mental construct:

Contact with person			
(client)		*Continuous thinking during Contact*	
Knowledge as before filtered through . . .	Self-care Concept	Nursing measures unknown	Outcome unknown

When clients came to me during the first year, I had to work in the self-care approach, no matter what specific concern had brought the person to my office. I had to start with the need expressed by the client, meet that need with professional nursing care, and at the same time incorporate the larger self-care concepts in dealing with the specific. An example was an elderly lady who came to my office and asked about burning on urination; she wondered if she could go on a hike the following day. In retrospect, I had this in my mind. When I examined her, I experienced the tension of caution built in over the years not to communicate any knowledge to the person. Yet I felt I had to "tell" her something. So, I blended the approaches.

Knowledge as before	*S-C Concept*	*N Measures*	*Outcome*
	Inspected the area (former pressures very heavy not to make diagnosis)	I safely laid out all alternatives, warning about chronic infections, safeguarding my replies. Aware that my perception of myself as a professional nurse was in a process of change, I straddled both self-concepts, and so (1) took refuge in "informing" the person about	Two days later called. All was OK. Had good time on hike.

medical complications (responsibility discharged); and (2) summoned courage to act on my knowledge from a beginning comprehension of judgment exercised within a range of normal—as opposed to a range of abnormal. Yes, she could go on a hike the following day. Moved from that to discussion of s-c assets and deficits.

By the spring of 1972, clients began coming to me saying, "I'm healthy; I'd like to stay that way; and I'd like you to make me healthier." So the clients began to supply me with the vocabulary that best expressed my concept of nursing practice, and which heretofore I had not been able to articulate fully. The mental construct now began to form in this way:

Contact with client		*Continuous thinking during contact*
Articulation of his self-care practices by the client.	His health goals	Nursing Measures given Use of Knowledge Base

Note that there is a shift in the position of the armamentarium of nursing action, in which I summon my knowledge to form a basis for judgment at the end, not the beginning. At this time I developed my definition of nursing practice: *Nursing is assisting the person in his self-care practices in regard to his state of health.* Every word is highly significant in terms of judgment-making on the part of the professional nurse.

Now, after five years in practice, I am secure in being able to describe the nursing approach that I take in the care of my clients and thus to differentiate clearly between medicine and nursing. I can defend the premise: A nurse can know as much as, and she can know more than, a physician, but she uses the knowledge toward goals of nursing care, which are different from the goals of medical care. Philosophically speaking, the formal object of medicine is disease, the diagnosis and treatment thereof; whereas the formal object of nursing is the person—body, mind and soul. In my conceptual frame of reference, I focus on the exercise of self-care agency in self-care practices in regard to a person's health state.

At this point my mental construct became:

Contact with Client   *Continuous thinking during contact*

| Client talk-ing | Identification of self-care practices by N with client | S-c assets and deficits by N | Therapeutic self-care demand by N | N measures by N | Outcome more predictable. |

Knowledge Base plus Experience

The concept was becoming so concrete in my mind that in 1974, in an article appearing in the *American Journal of Nursing*, I was able to state: "I now view medical care as a part of nursing care, and isn't that a switch?"

chapter three

The initiation
of change:
establishing the practice

There is perhaps no single experience in my life that can be pinpointed as the impetus for my decision to open an independent nursing practice. I would have to say, however, that the movement began, albeit subconsciously, almost 30 years ago. During those years various experiences were exerting subtle influences that would rise to the surface during the late 1960s.

I had no way of knowing it then, of course, but my secondary and my baccalaureate education were preparing me in a unique way for the action I was to take in 1971. When I was a student at Mount de Sales Academy and later at Notre Dame College, I was interested in literature, writing and languages. In college I majored in French, minored in Spanish, and had a total of seven years of Latin and two of Greek. Courses in philosophy, including logic, psychology, criteriology and metaphysics equipped me to reason in an orderly fashion, according to the dictates of the science of thought. Through the study of poetry, literature and languages, I learned the surpassing beauty of words, and I viewed the human experience of centuries through the study of the classics. With this background, it was natural for me to resist taking my subsequent training in nursing at face value and to view it critically; also, it was natural for me to want to view the totality of a situation, or of a person, and to act accordingly. I believe that these mental sets were instrumental in shaping my subsequent actions as a professional nurse.

I decided to become a nurse because, after graduation from college in 1943, I wanted to do something for my country during World War II. Nursing offered a ladylike pursuit with unquestioned benefits to my country, so in 1944 I entered the Catholic University of America School of Nursing in Washington, D.C. I received my BSN in 1946 and continued with my studies, earning a BSNE in 1947 and an MSNE in 1953.

Immediately after graduation I began to teach nursing. To gain experience in the practice of nursing I would, during the evening, take care of the patients assigned to my students for the following morning. I also worked part time in a physician's office. In 1953–54 I was supervisor-instructor at the Johns Hopkins School of Nursing in Baltimore, while on leave from the Catholic University of America, and from 1947–59 I taught the fundamentals of nursing and medical-surgical nursing at Catholic University.

It was not long after I began to teach nursing that I started to feel frustration. When I was teaching professional nurses in the BSRN program, the content for which I was responsible consisted of topics such as "The Professional Nurse in Modern Society," "Principles of Management," and a "Clinical Practicum." But POSDCORB* was not "nursing," and changes in society affecting the field of nursing could not be considered "nursing." How do you teach professional registered nurses content that is called "nursing," I would ask myself, when in reality it was a rehashing of the material they had already learned in their three-year diploma programs? The quality of the teachers in general determined the learning, of course, but basically the students already understood the content. If what they had learned in their basic three-year programs was not adequate, why were they practicing nursing? Why did they

---

* Acronym used in management literature. It stands for planning, organizing, staffing, directing, coordinating, reporting, budgeting. Source: Forest W. Horton, Jr., *Reference Guide to Advanced Management Methods* (New York: American Management Assoc., Inc., 1972), p. 135.

have licenses? If the baccalaureate program was going to offer something of an academic nature in nursing, then it could hardly concentrate on remedying poor organization of nursing activities or sloppy procedural techniques; nor could it introduce advances in medical care and the related technology. Under these educational circumstances, I felt the best I could offer was to develop in the student an acceptance of the responsibility that any professional person has to define the nature of his or her profession (in this case, nursing) and to emphasize the premise that is the foundation of the nursing profession—that a professional nurse must be known by the care she gives to the person for whom she is caring.

After additional study of cardiovascular nursing at the University of Minnesota in 1959, I became the director of the only program then available in the nation—located at Catholic University—which offered a course of study leading to a master's degree in cardiovascular nursing. During this period, in the 1960s, I was a member of a committee of faculty members investigating the development of a nursing model. In this committee, we worked with the concept of self-care as described by Dorothea Orem in her book *Nursing: Concepts of Practice.* I gained many insights into the intricacies of the problem of identifying a concept of nursing that is comprehensive, concise, consistent, cohesive and complete—traits that must apply to any proposed concept. Simultaneously, my disenchantment with the substance of the "nursing" I was teaching and the lack of scientific research into a valid basis for acting to achieve a *nursing* goal thrust me into an enigmatical intellectual orbit. When, for example, I heard the frequently asked question "What is new in cardiovascular nursing?" I would reply, "Nothing. We still take blood pressures standing up, for instance. If we stood on our heads to take blood pressures, that would be new. But all the new knowledge is in the fields of bioengineering, physiology, physics and chemistry. Medicine has applied it, but nursing sits on it." I would go on to explain that the nurse is exposed to the application of that knowledge to a pathological state and to its

---

* Dorothea Orem, *Nursing: Concepts of Practice* (New York: McGraw-Hill Book Company, 1971).

use in explaining something possibly abnormal; and it is from this standpoint that she gains new knowledge and goes on to take action in light of that knowledge. The need for monitoring blood gases and the administration of drugs in acute and chronic conditions of the medical state comprised the bulk of the content in the nursing literature. Invariably, the end product of learning was the mastery of a technique, such as the reading of an electrocardiogram—and this bore the label "nursing." The result of this situation was that any decision was a medical decision and any act a medical act, because the goal was a medical one. I was tormented by the conspicuous absence of criteria that would assure the person performing the act—the nurse—that the judgment she was called upon to make was in reality "nursing." I gave assignments to the graduate students that required them to identify a nursing goal when they were in the coronary care unit, when they were in the recovery room caring for a person who had undergone open heart surgery, when they were helping a person with hypertension or with a peripheral vascular ulcer, and when they were performing other tasks that required the new knowledge that the master's program was supplying them. They could not do this, and neither could I. All that could be identified was a medical goal. To use one's judgment was to make a medical judgment.

New Knowledge ——— New Tasks ——— For What Purpose?

This was the dilemma in nursing as I saw it.

What emerged was concrete and clear to me. Either the nurse had to learn in a medical school what the physician learned, so that the judgment would be a solid medical one leaving no doubt in the mind of the nurse, or the nurse needed to learn far less—if merely carrying out an ordered technique or procedure was the reason for her presence. In neither proposition could I find assurance that the end result would be "nursing." Just because a nurse carries out an action, that action does not automatically become nursing. The nebulousness about what nursing consisted of continued to underscore the polarity I felt between what nurses did—and called "nursing"—and what could be indisputably, objectively and defensibly identified as *nursing.* Because the medical needs of the patients determined the parameters of nursing care, because nursing was always confined within the parameters of medicine, I felt that the knowledge was either unnecessary or insufficient; there seemed to be no middle ground in terms of action on the part of the nurse.

In a way, the more I learned, the more frustration I experienced. Each time I tried to apply the knowledge I had acquired to the actual practice of nursing I became more aware that I was not free to use it. I also became conscious of another disturbing fact—the fact that the preferences of individual physicians had to be constantly borne in mind and observed in regard to the care of an individual patient. This fact further supported my contention that I was engaged not so much in nursing as in meticulously carrying out measures assuring a *medical* outcome, measures concerned with the *medical* state of the patient—a worthwhile goal, of course, but not a *nursing* goal. When the medical regimen prescribed by some physicians was in direct conflict with validated data to be observed in the care of patients with cardiovascular disease, I in turn was torn by an intolerable conflict—the conflict between what I wanted to do, based on fact, and what I had to do, based on a physician's order. I developed what I call "intellectual allergy," which may best be portrayed in this fashion:

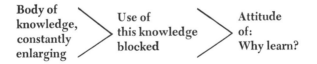

Body of knowledge, constantly enlarging > Use of this knowledge blocked > Attitude of: Why learn?

In the traditional setting, there was no way out of a multitude of frustrating situations. For example, a physician would tell his patient that he was giving her potassium "to clear out the impurities in the blood," and the patient would ask me, "What does that mean—what impurities?" In the traditional setting of nursing, however, I was powerless to share my knowledge with the patient to relieve her anxieties. I once had a patient who was receiving nitrogen mustard, and I was attempting to teach a nursing student about the case by going over the chart with her. Suddenly the physician snatched the chart from my hands and said, "What are you doing, talking about that?

That's none of your concern. Just teach those students to give bedpans and then to remove them." In situations such as those, in which knowledge was expected of the nurse by the *patient* and no knowledge was expected of the nurse by the *physician,* the frustration was overwhelming. I remember pacing the hall outside my office in the hospital after that humiliating episode, trying to rid myself of my anger, bewilderment and discouragement. Somehow, the patients were the losers if I was unable to contact them and help them. Another example of illogical procedure was the requirement that even when a nurse knew the obvious action to take to help a patient, she must wait until an "order" could be obtained. For example, a patient's bladder might be so distended with urine that he would be in a great deal of pain. There would be no reason why he could not be catheterized, an accepted method of emptying the bladder at that time. Yet an hour or more would elapse before the "order" could be obtained.

To me the choice was becoming clear—it was either to stay in nursing in the traditional settings and keep the professional nursing I longed to practice in shackles, or to enter a new setting in which I would be free to help people as a professional nurse. I had also ascertained at this time that the lay person was much more informed about medical matters than seemed to be recognized by the physicians of the day. Furthermore, I realized that lay persons were perplexed about how to communicate to the physician what they knew objectively and also about how to put this together with what they and only they knew about themselves and their health state.

At this point in the development of my concept of nursing, I was struggling with the algebraic equivalent of terms of a proposition that could be structured in this way:

Knowns

Knowledge (on part of nurse)
Knowledge (on part of person)   About *disease* of the person
Knowledge (on part of person)   About his *usual health state*

Action (on part of physician)
Action (on part of person)   In regard to *medical state*
Action (on part of nurse)

Unknowns
Knowledge (on part of nurse) about *person's usual health state*
Action (on part of nurse) in regard to *person's usual health state*

Conclusions:
Find out the usual health state of individual. Take action in light of both sets of knowledge.

Eureka! Person plus knowledge: Nurse plus knowledge: Person plus action: Nurse plus action. Therefore: Nurse must learn what knowledge the person has, before nursing care can be given. Further, since the person with knowledge sometimes needs help in the application of this knowledge (proof of this need can be found in nursing literature over the decades), a further postulation was formed.

Knowns
Action (on part of person) is determined by motivation.
Motivation is determined by goal sought.
Therefore, action is determined by goal sought.
Therefore: Nurse must know goal of person before nursing care can be
   given.

It was clear to me why I could not give professional nursing care in the traditional settings. It was as impossible for me to give nursing care in the presence of so many unknowns as it is impossible to say when you will arrive at a destination when you know neither the point of departure nor the mode of travel. The essence of nursing cannot be captured when the substance of the action the nurse is taking is obviously movement directed toward a goal in another field—for it is inevitable that changes in the other field will determine what actions the person called "nurse" will take, and that these actions will become part of the content called "nursing." The illogic was apparent; two professions cannot have the same goals. Either nursing is a profession—and accordingly must have goals of its own—or it is not a profession.

My thoughts about nursing as a profession were crystallizing. Armed with the embryonic concept of self-care in terms of health, and beginning to understand the perspective of myself as an extension of the client, I chose a position in a setting that I thought would enable me to practice nursing within this newly articulated concept. The position I took was that of night charge nurse in a nursing home. There I would be able to care for individuals who were not in an acute medical state and who were in that institution for nursing care. I could use the knowledge I had acquired over the years to a far greater degree than I had ever been able to use it. There was a clearer delineation of the difference between nursing and medicine in this setting, and I had my own knowledge on which to base my actions. So at one point I was able to write on one patient's chart, with no misgivings or doubts, the following words. "Because the physician is interfering with my nursing care, I will no longer take responsibility for the care of this resident." (See Chapter 7, page 121 for details of this situation.)

It was at this time that I sensed that the goal of being in independent practice was within reach. During the previous 22 years, I had commented from time to time about opening an independent nursing office, but the time, place and method were unknown. I remember specifically saying to the graduate students in the cardiovascular nursing program that someday I would have my own office. Later, they told me they had no idea of what I was talking about; "it bollixed our minds," they said. Now, it was all becoming clearer in my own mind. After seven months in the nursing home, I felt I could consider one of the various academic positions which would put me into the mainstream of nursing education again and allow me the flexibility to plan my course of action for an independent practice. I chose to join the faculty of the Georgetown University School of Nursing, beginning in June 1970. The curriculum was being revised, the core of the changes being the integration of the self-care concept of nursing throughout the four years of the program. Later that summer, I knew I would be in independent practice by the following year, but the place and procedure were still nebulous. I was certain of one thing, however. I knew I could articulate the concept of self-care in nursing to a degree that would enable me to practice nursing and to be sure I was not practicing medicine. In retrospect, when I picked up the phone in March, 1971, and began to inquire about office space, I can recall no specific reason for doing so precisely at that moment. Except that I knew I was ready.

I was ready, I felt, to help people as a professional nurse. My background included a liberal arts education, nursing degrees, teacher preparation and years of teaching and practicing nursing. I was convinced that nursing was unique and that it could be offered to the people just as any other profession could. Before attending to the details of opening my office, however, I had to take account of the basic criteria that indicate to the public that a service is professional, and I had to make certain that my practice would meet those criteria. Those criteria and their application to the traditional practice of nursing may be summarized as follows:

Any Profession	*Practice of Nursing (Traditional)*
1. *Availability:* knowledge by the public that there are offices out of which the professional service is dispensed	No knowledge by public of offices out of which professional nursing is given
2. *Accessibility:* contact by phone or letter for appointment	No contact for appointment for professional nursing services
3. *Accuracy:* members of the profession use the latest developments in the field, learned through data collection, results of lab tests, precedent cases, experimental design, etc.	Consists of implementation of scientific advances of other fields; few studies of the intrinsic nature of nursing
4. *Accountability:* constant communication between client and professional until a terminus is reached	Communication has been obscure, indirect and erratic, usually limited as part of contact with a physician, hospital, other nurses, etc.
5. *Autonomy:* initial direction determined by the professional; initial decision-making, sustained implementation of judgments, evaluation of results, termination, analysis of effectiveness	Initiation, continuation and termination of action dependent upon someone else, such as a physician, hospital, etc.

In addition to those, I set forth five criteria specifically relating to my practice. I decided that (1) I had to be completely alone in my practice; (2) I had to subsidize my own office; (3) I had to establish a fee for services; (4) I had to be a generalist; and (5) I had to practice within the self-care concept of nursing.

Operating alone in my practice would enable me to maintain complete control and to direct the course of endeavor. This would satisfy the requirements for autonomy and accountability. In addition, offering my services in a practice alone would make clear to the public exactly what kind of services were being offered—a professional nurse in independent practice as opposed to, for example, a nurse assisting in the medical setting of a clinic or hospital. Thus, my practice would have availability and accessibility. A person could call on me directly for nursing, instead of having to become ill and seek the services of a physician in order to have fleeting contact with a nurse functioning as part of the medical regime. Further, subsidizing my own office would guarantee no policy controls, again ensuring that I would have the autonomy to direct the course of endeavor in the best interests of my clients.

Establishing a fee for services was a method of recognition of services rendered, a barometer for the assessment of the public need for such services, and a means of evaluating my own effectiveness. In establishing the fee, it seemed vital to choose a figure that was small enough to assure that the cost would not preclude persons from seeking my nursing care in the first place, and to assure further that it could not be seen by the client as a reason for not returning to me for nursing care. Thus, if clients whose needs indicated sustained nursing care did not return, I could know that the reason was probably their view of the nature of the nursing care they had received and of the way they thought it had helped them.

The criterion of accuracy in any profession depends on the professional person's knowledge of his field, for it is on this that he bases his judgment and art of practice. The substantive nature of other professions is well identified and known by all members. The substantive nature of a given profession can be observed as it is applied by all of the generalists in the field; and it is the point of departure for all of the specialists in the field. In nursing, however, the substantive nature of the field has never been fully identified, so the term "general nursing" does not convey a circumscribed notion, as the terms "general medicine" or "general law" do. I felt that I had to start with the identification of nursing needs *generally* as presented by clients, so I chose to practice as a generalist nurse. It is my position that we have not gathered information on nursing needs from people, but have defined the needs of people (patients) ourselves because they possessed medical needs (medical-surgical, obstetrical, pediatric conditions, etc.). Taking the breadth of the meaning of the self-care concept in health states, I decided to give full rein to the expression of needs by persons as *they* saw those needs. (After general nursing has been defined and mastered, criteria of accuracy can be set up and professional expertise measured against them. The nursing literature should begin to change as the general nature of nursing is identified through the application of a concept to the practice of nursing. The curricula of schools of nursing should then change to reflect the developed and developing body of knowledge. This, in turn, will foster an increased awareness by the public of the substantive nature of nursing.)

With the criteria of professionalism and my own conditions of practice in mind, I picked up the telephone one afternoon in March, 1971, called a realtor and inquired about office space. He quoted a figure for the rent on two rooms, and I remember deciding it was too high. I then looked in the Yellow Pages for another Maryland realtor and my eye was caught by one in College Park, Maryland, a city of about 26,000, approximately 15 miles outside of Washington, D.C., but close to my own apartment. I called, and the realtor told me he had a small building that I could rent for the amount the first realtor had quoted for only two rooms. That afternoon I drove over to look at it and knew immediately that it would be my first office. I returned with a friend a few days later, and without further ado I rented the building. I had the choice of renting only one story or one or two rooms, and I decided to rent the entire building. It was important, I reasoned, that I avoid the risk of having tenants in the remaining offices who might possibly jeopardize the image of a professional nurse in independent practice. Also, I had no way of knowing which direction my practice would take. Would groups approach me for nursing care? Would I need the other rooms? It seemed better to have too much room than not enough.

The building was located in a lower-middle-income residential area, an important factor, since I did not want the location to define the practice, as a ghetto or rural site would tend to do. The building was a two-story wood frame house that had been altered for office use by means of paneling and doors. It had a front porch, a small front lawn and two gas lamps that were still operable. And it was within my budget— $325.00 a month for rent. Later, I found that my additional monthly payments amounted to approximately $55 to the gas and light company, $20 to the electric company, and $35 to the telephone company.

Inside the building, I strove to keep the office as homelike as possible and to avoid the atmosphere of a medical setting. Because nursing is different from medicine, it was important that I show my clients an atmosphere that was different from a medical one. If a person walked in my door and immediately encountered the same white and stainless steel environment he saw when he visited his physician, he would see my nursing in the medical context. Accordingly, the environment in my office had to be consonant with the substance of what I had formulated as my concept of what I would be doing as a professional nurse—providing the opportunity for a client to talk, for me to listen to his needs as he saw them, and then for me to choose what I needed to help that client in view of these needs. Because I did not wish to influence the direction of the client's needs through the appearance of the setting, I kept the office bare of equipment, except for a desk and file cabinet in one corner. Thus, the room in which the client and I met was in essence a living room. The client sat on a small sofa, and I drew up one of two armchairs to face him, or I sat beside him at an oblique angle as he sat in one of the chairs. I never sat behind a desk when I was with a client. And I never wore a uniform of any kind.

In an adjoining room, I stored the few items which would be necessary for minor first aid situations. The items I had purchased were those that any home first aid kit would contain: Band-Aids, alcohol, merthiolate, cotton balls, four by fours and adhesive tape. In a closet in the same room I kept a stethoscope and a blood pressure cuff. (Later, I purchased an EKG unit, otoscope and ophthalmoscope.)

In general, I knew what I was trying to communicate to the persons who would seek my services, and I wanted my office to communicate this message, too—"I can give you nursing care, and it is not second-rate medical care or substitute medicine."

This point was in my mind, too, when I called to establish contact with a laboratory. I thought that there might be instances in which a client would want to know his blood picture or urinalysis findings from time to time, as part of his knowledge of his total health state. So in the fall of 1971 I called the most prestigious laboratory in the District of Columbia. The lay person who talked with me about my request for occasional service was enthusiastic about my idea of practice, and said he felt that there would be no reason why I could not send specimens to that laboratory. However, as a matter of procedure, he said, he would check with the physician in charge of the laboratory and call me back. When he called the next morning, there was a changed note in his voice (it was almost apologetic) and he indicated that the physician in charge wanted to ask me a few questions. When I spoke with the physician, the conversation went like this:

"Yes, Miss Kinlein, Mr. ——— told me about your request, and I would just like to find out one or two things. Who is the doctor you are working with?"

"There is no doctor."

"No doctor? Then how can you do anything?"

I explained that I would be practicing nursing according to a concept of nursing which insured that I would be practicing nursing and not medicine.

"Well, who will read these reports and interpret them?"

"I will."

His voice became authoritative. "But you can't do that. A doctor is required to do that."

"Not really. In the hospital, the nurse always reads and interprets the lab reports before she calls a physician, to see if it is necessary to call the physician."

"That's different."

"No. I don't think so."

"Well, this puts a different light on the matter of having laboratory work done here at this laboratory."

I had nothing more to lose, so I tried to indicate the scope of my work with clients—"I am saving up for an electrocardiograph so I can take EKGs."

"*What?* Well, who would interpret those?"

"I will."

"Oh, now you can't do *that*. That's clearly making a diagnosis. Only a physician can read an EKG and make a diagnosis. Not a nurse or anybody else." He was becoming quite angry.

"You know, Dr. ———," I said very softly, "I am thinking about a session of the American Heart Association at which a cardiologist said in his address, 'If any physician makes a diagnosis from an electrocardiogram, he ought to go back to medical school.'" There was a brief silence.

He continued, "I have built this laboratory to the point where it has the highest regard by the medical world for accuracy and integrity, and I want to keep it that way. Why, when the abortion clinic in the next block asked me to do their lab work, I refused, and there were *physicians* there. But it was against my principles."

I responded, again softly, but with a sense of having been insulted—"I know how prestigious your laboratory is and how much you are respected in the District. That is why I called you first. And it is so good to hear someone standing by his principles in today's society. I would like to compliment you."

"Yes," he said, pleased with my compliment. "So if I refused to do their work, you see I can't accept yours under the circumstances."

We concluded the conversation. The next four calls to other laboratories in the metropolitan area were also fruitless because there was no doctor working with me.

Finally, the sixth laboratory I called responded affirmatively. I shall always be grateful to Dr. Matta of the McCoy, Morales, Garcia, and Matta laboratory group. I explained my practice, and he said, "I see no reason why such an arrangement cannot be made. I think it is a fine thing you have done."

The fact that the public, too, had a structured idea of nursing was evidenced by the comments of the various persons who came to my office in the early days of my practice. The telephone man wanted to know if it was "going to be a nursery." Another workman said, "Oh, I know, it's going to be a registry for nurses." The inspector for the county department of licenses and permits came to inspect the office to see if it met the code for an office of its type. "What shall I look for?" he asked me. "This is so different, so new—a nurse having her own office just like a doctor or lawyer. I just can't think what I should be looking for and asking about." An eight-year-old boy who came to ask me if I had seen his lost puppy looked around and asked me where the beds with the sick people were. "Are you really a nurse?" he asked. "You don't have a white uniform on!" He went on to say, "Could I come to you for this cut on my head? (showing it to me). That's where my sister hit me with a rock. And here on my chest my pet rabbit scratched me." He looked around the office, asked me again to let him know if I saw his dog, talked a little more about some of the children in the neighborhood and then left.

"What should I have wrong with me that would cause me to come to you? Why should I come to you?" were questions that reporters and other lay persons would ask. I would reply, "You would come to me if you thought you needed a professional nurse." "How would people know they need to come to a nurse?" was another question. Gradually, I found myself responding, "I would hope that you would have nothing wrong with you, and I would want to help you maintain your health state through good self-care practices on a daily basis."

Nursing colleagues, too, would ask me exactly what I would be doing. My response was candid. "I don't know. It depends on what my clients' needs will be." I had no idea exactly what needs would be presented to me. And to attempt to estimate the needs in advance would have been contrary to my concept of nursing. A prior expectation or judgment of a need on my part would have limited my ability to "hear" the needs as expressed by the client, and thus would have limited the effectiveness of my nursing.

When my nursing colleagues asked if I could legally open an independent nursing practice, I was surprised. The idea in my mind was so solid that I had never doubted its legality. A greatly trusted colleague said, "Lucille, don't touch a person until you have seen a lawyer," and I was shaken by her comment. I had already signed the lease for my office, but because of my great respect for her, I took her advice. Another nursing colleague had recommended that, if I were going to see a lawyer, I consult the attorney who represented the District of Columbia Nursing Association, because of his familiarity with nursing. I went to his office and told him of my plans. "What does it mean? What will you be doing?" he asked. I explained my self-care concept of nursing and told him that I would not diagnose or treat illness because that is the essence of the practice of medicine. I explained that I did not yet know exactly what needs would be presented to me, but that I would be giving people nursing care defined in terms of self-care—helping a person physically and psychologically through an illness, or before an illness or after recovery. When he asked if I would give a person medication, I explained that I would administer only medication already prescribed by a physician, such as insulin injections, as any other nurse could do. "What will the people come to you for?" he asked. I replied, "I don't know. That's what I shall find out. I know that I know nursing. What I am asking you is this—from a legal standpoint, as a professional person opening an office, is there any reason I cannot open this nursing practice?" The lawyer pulled out the appropriate volume of the Maryland Code from his bookshelves and read aloud the Nurse-Practice Act for Maryland, which I had memorized by that time. I was already licensed to practice nursing in Maryland and in the District of Columbia, and I knew that I would operate my independent practice within the boundaries of the law he read to me. I knew that I was free to start my practice, and the lawyer confirmed this. He concluded that there was prima facie evidence that it was appropriate for me to start my own practice, and he saw no legal reason why I should not.

Another matter deserving attention before I could open my practice was the whole question of nursing care in the case of an emergency. I was aware that I might be confronted with a situation in which someone had sustained an injury or had been stricken with an illness of an acute nature requiring emergency care. My conceptual basis for handling such a situation was formulated this way:

First, most people know that they should call an ambulance or get to a hospital emergency room in the case of an accident. Newspapers and television have publicized the work of rescue workers, emergency squads, trauma centers and the like. I recall a question from one physician in an audience that I was addressing after the opening of my office. He asked, if a person came to my office with an open fracture of the leg, in a state of unconsciousness, with breathing difficulties, what I would do in the treatment of that person? I replied that the person would never have been brought to my office, that he would have been taken to an emergency room. I added that he would not even have been taken to the office of the physician who asked the question. The physician's comment was, "Touché."

In addition, many persons know first aid measures and are not at all reluctant to apply their knowledge in an emergency. Cardio-pulmonary resuscitation, as well as other first aid measures, is being taught in grade schools in various states in the nation. And some restaurants have posted in conspicuous spots the currently favored procedure of removing food that is blocking the trachea.

However, because there was an auto repair shop next to my office, and because of the many children in the neighborhood, I considered the possibility of being confronted with an emergency situation. So I briefed myself on all types of injuries and the various first aid measures for them. (I even bought a book entitled *Emergency War Measures*. I thought I might find an obscurely placed gem, the principle of which might apply in the instance of, for example, a crushed chest caused by the weight of a car which had fallen when the jack slipped.) On the corner of my desk I pasted the telephone number of the fire department located across the street from the auto repair shop. As I attempted to identify where the line existed between first aid and first-line medical therapy, the distinction became more and more obvious. I worked through this concept in regard to emergency situations:

The three elements that should be present on the part of the person who helps are: (1) knowledge, (2) judgment, (3) action—which may be initiated to prevent action by someone else.

Situation 1—Physician

A physician is called and responds to the needs of the person who is sick, injured or unconscious. He takes measures that are identified in the literature as first aid measures.

Situation 1—Nurse

An attempt is made to summon a physician, but none is available. A professional nurse is summoned and takes the same measures that the physician would take in an identical situation.

Situation 1—Lay person

Neither a physician nor a nurse is available. A lay person responds to the need and takes the same measures that the physician and nurse would take in identical situations.

Was first aid rendered in all three circumstances? The answer would have to be yes. On the other hand, if all three individuals were present in another situation, several ramifications emerge.

Situation 2—P, N, and L

If the signs and symptoms can be objectified so that they are readily apparent, would more experience and more recent exposure to emergency situations on the part of the lay person, as compared to that of the physician and nurse, be recognized as being more helpful to the person needing help? Would the doctor and the nurse stand aside and let the lay person administer first aid?

I felt satisfied that I would be secure in rendering first aid; I knew that I could explain why I did not do more, if the situation arose in which I was challenged. For myself, I had drawn the line between first aid and first-line medical care and was secure about the possibility of an emergency situation requiring first aid. After first aid, any action would constitute medical therapy. To date, no emergency situation of this kind has ever presented itself in my practice.

The next step was to make my professional nursing services available. Because of my concept of professional nursing, and because I believed that the nursing needs of people had not been identified, it was imperative that nothing be done to induce lay persons to seek my services. In the minds of the public, nursing was an adjunct to medicine, and any time they approached a nurse for care, or a nurse approached them to give care, the need had flowed from the medical condition of the person; hence, to assume that the stated need was a nursing need simply because it was presented to a nurse was erroneous. Therefore, in my practice I wanted to identify in as scientific a manner as possible what nursing needs were. I had to strip away everything that might influence the individual to seek my services. The conditions that I set up were that the person would have to phone me for an appointment (at which time he would become my client), come to see me or ask me to make a house call, and from that point on, I would be giving him nursing care. Further, I had to be visible in the community in the acceptable fashion of a professional person, and I decided that a shingle would be an acceptable method. It hung from one of the gas lamps and read, "M. Lucille Kinlein, R.N." Only when my colleagues asked me what I practiced *as* did I call myself an "independent nurse practitioner." The title "pediatric nurse practitioner" was already in the nursing vocabulary at that time, in 1971. Later, the literature in the nursing field, especially during the years 1973–1975, abounded with articles about the developing movement of the "nurse practitioner." In all instances, I found in that movement the same point of departure as in medicine, namely, a frame of reference of pathology; and in most instances there was the need for contact with a physician to varying degrees. I became concerned, therefore, that the title "nurse practitioner" would make me appear to be cast in the same mold. So it behooved me to find another title for myself. I chose "independent generalist nurse." (When I opened my second office in Bowie, Maryland, in the fall of 1975, I used that title for the plaque on the door. It reads, "M. Lucille Kinlein, R.N.," and beneath that, "Independent Generalist Nurse." I had the plaque on the door of my Hyattsville office, to which I moved in 1974, changed to read the same.)

The shingle for my first office was to have a short life. It was stolen from the lamp post, and when I had another one made and placed it inside a front window, someone broke the glass and took the replacement. I did not replace the second shingle, but by that time I was receiving clients from the recommendations of others. In fact, the only person who came to my office because she saw the shingle was a young girl who wanted to have her ears pierced. I explained that I could not pierce her ears and warned her about the possibility of infection in the ear lobe after such a procedure. I then gave her the names of some physicians in the area who do pierce ears. I refer to her as a person and not as a client because obviously she did not become my client.

Another method of making my nursing services available was to send out announcements of the opening of the office. I had 200 printed, but in the end I sent only 18 of them. Protocol demanded that the American Nurse's Association receive one, as well as the D.C. Board of Nurse Examiners. I also sent announcements to the American Medical Association, to each of the directors of nursing service in the area hospitals, to each of the deans of the university schools of nursing in the area, and to the D.C. Nurse's Association and the D.C. League for Nursing. I decided to send only those. I was very cautious about "advertising" myself. I wanted people to come to me because they recognized their need for a nurse. So it seemed to me that the shingle and word-of-mouth recommendations would have to suffice.

I sat back and waited for my first client to come. It is especially gratifying—indeed a case of poetic justice —that my first client was a professional nurse. She came to me at the recommendation of another professional nurse, Loretta Nowakowski, a member of the Georgetown University faculty. My first client came on August 20, 1971, at 7 P.M., and presented me with the first nursing needs to be met in my independent practice. She wanted to discuss a health situation affecting her family. Her mother, who was suffering from bronchial pneumonia, had been caring for her father, who had Parkinson's disease and had suffered a stroke. The client was concerned that her mother catered too much to her father and was jeopardizing her own health further. The client indicated that she would feel guilty about putting her father in a nursing home, and yet eventually expressed that that was exactly what she really wanted to do. As she explained the physical and emotional factors involved, I was able to view the situation in its entirety, and at the same time she was able to see her own feelings more clearly. The nursing care measures that were established were that:

1. I would visit her mother and her father to gain a more complete picture of the physical and mental state of each one.
2. I would continue to follow through on the implementation of the plan that would be formulated after I had given initial care to her parents.
3. I would gather nursing home information so that it would be ready when it was needed.

Her mother and father became clients number 2 and number 3 in my practice. It seemed especially fitting that in my first client situation the needs expressed were consonant with the professional nursing I longed to give—learning the physical, emotional and spiritual factors that were affecting the health maintenance of a person, and of others close to her, and helping the persons involved to implement effective self-care measures to cope with a stressful situation. This family remained as steady clients until their needs were met. My practice grew quickly and by October included 19 clients, 16 of whom returned more than once for continued nursing care.

In addition to word of-mouth recommendations, the public was made aware of my practice through publicity in the media. A friend of mine had called *The Washington Star* and told reporter Joy Billington about my practice, and she wrote the first article about me. The article was picked up from the *New York Times* wire service by other papers, and soon I received clippings of stories applauding the endeavor from newspapers all over the country, sent by friends, former students and strangers. Other newspapers, television and radio stations and *Time* magazine covered the story as well. Fortunately, the clients who came to me as a result of this publicity recommended me to others, and most of my clients subsequently came because of word-of-mouth recommendations.

Client number 8 also stands out in my mind because the nature of his needs led me, for the first time, to contact a physician about a client. A man who had done some cleaning for me called one week and requested an appointment to discuss an impotence problem. After we discussed the problem and I answered his questions, I found it necessary to suggest that he see a physician. After a physician had been selected by both of us, I wrote to the doctor and summarized the points I thought would be significant, so that he would have a more complete picture of my client's health state. I had no way of knowing what the physician's reaction would be. Years of uncertainty had conditioned me to wonder, Would he merely throw the letter away? Would he telephone irately? In the event that he called, I formulated in advance what my response would be. The outcome was gratifying, however. The physician wrote to me giving me the details of his medical examination and diagnosis and thanked me for allowing him "to be of help." We continued to correspond about my client, and later I wrote to him, "Cognizant of the historical significance of the opening of the first office by a nurse to engage in the practice of nursing, I am especially pleased that my eighth client became a patient receiving your medical care. He was the first in my practice for whom a medical referral was necessary. . . . A highly satisfactory relationship has set a desirable precedent that should be followed in similar situations in the future. I look forward to our continued relationship and thank you for your assistance in the care of (my client)."

When one recalls the early days of a practice, time becomes relative. In my practice, scarcely five years old, were the early days in 1971 or 1972? Were the early days in 1973, or in 1974, when the practice seemed to mushroom? The rapidity with which the practice has grown (I now have about 800 clients) has precluded statistical analysis in percentages of growth over the years. When speaking, then, of the early clients, I shall confine the time period to the first two years, May 1971 to May 1973.

Some of the clients who first came to me had difficulty understanding that I was not practicing in affiliation with physicians. They extended compliments about the knowledge of nurses and the fact that they often have to make decisions about the medical state of patients in the traditional settings. They further commented that "they (nurses) do all the work and doctors get all the credit," and that people would rather go to nurses anyway because they are so understanding about the person and his problem. Very carefully I would accept their compliments and after a few more were given, I would explain as succinctly as possible that, while I use the knowledge I have, I use it in a different way than doctors do; that my goal is different from that of the doctors; and that I am an extension of the person rather than an extension of the physician. I would never accept the comment that nurses are "doing this" because the doctors are so busy.

On the other hand, there were clients who from the beginning knew that I was offering a different type of care in the health system. "You are different from doctors and from the nurses I know," one client said. "I think nursing care is different from medical care, and it could not be seen until someone did what you did. You should have a different title, though. It is more than the traditional, yet it includes the traditional. It is different. I know when I need you, and I know when I need a doctor. We have to get a different title for you so people will know all you can do for them."

Sometimes I am asked whether I encountered any hypochondriacs in my practice, or even if the majority of my clients had hypochondriacal tendencies. My response was and still is, even in retrospect, an emphatic no. I say "in retrospect" because it is possible that in the initial excitement of being in practice, of building my own enterprise, I could have misread some of the early clients and their expression of needs. But, indeed, the early clients are etched in my memory in a very special way. When I look back at the notes taken during the health history phase of an appointment, I can fill in much about the client that was not written. As my technique of taking the health history has improved, my records have become more complete and the memory less strained. As a matter of fact, the variety of needs that I encountered in the early days of the practice gave me insight into what was to come as I continued with my care. After I had been in practice a year or so, categories of client needs could be identified this way:

Category 1—under a doctor's care, satisfied; he can't help me now; I need a nurse.

Category 2—not under a doctor's care; which doctor should I see?

Category 3—should I see a doctor? I need to get my allergy shot; should I have the brain scan and other tests?

In fact, at no time during any speaking engagement was I unable to answer the question "What would you do if . . . ?" Invariably, I was able to say, "Well, just yesterday, or last week, a client came to my office with just this problem. . . ." And, in response to questions such as, "Have you had any children as clients . . . or men . . . or pregnant women . . . or families . . . or members of minority groups . . . ?" I was always able to answer yes.

It was not easy, in those early days, to change my orientation from what I had been taught in nursing. Every time I advised a client about anything, there was a terrible nagging feeling, similar to what I would have felt in the traditional setting if I had given a medication for which there was no "order." The pressure would be compounded by the empathic feelings that accompanied giving a person an aspirin for a headache—relief for the patient, which made me feel competent and professional, yet which burdened me, as a nurse, for I knew that I was subjecting myself to the criticism of my fellow nurses. Added to all this were the conflicting responses of physicians. One doctor, upon learning that his patient had been given an aspirin, would be very irate; a resident would have applauded the action. The result was a schizophrenic, stress-producing situation for the nurse. Each nurse can add to the lengthy list of such situations, which were part of the everyday routine in most hospitals—the ultimate being the example of a licensed practical nurse who, in an emergency situation, in the absence of a physician or professional nurse, inserted an endo-tracheal tube in a patient on a respiratory unit. The action was supported enthusiastically by the resident, denounced by the attending physician, and supported by some nurses and not by others.

The terrible pressure of having to make judgments and decisions even within the framework of nursing cannot be minimized. In the first year of the practice, I experienced a physiological reaction with symptoms of acute stress in almost every instance—not knowing whether my care would be effective, having to wait until I heard from the client (I could not merely walk down the hall to see if the medicine had worked, as a nurse in a hospital setting could do), wondering if new clients would keep their appointments and if the old ones would return. There was a terrible Silence Out There, with no colleagues to fall back on, no established body of knowledge about nursing in an independent practice to build on —as doctors or lawyers have in their fields—no articles in the nursing journals offering me the benefit of others' experiences as independent practitioners. During 1971–72, expressions of need by my clients were followed by my imparting my knowledge to them and adding a tenuously worded recommendation about the course of action they should pursue. The crutch "probably it would be better if you consulted a doctor to reassure yourself" was clearly used to assure myself and stated because it was part of my traditional nursing lessons. Caution was the byword, and time from month to month was my ally.

Always heavy on my mind in the early days, too, was an awareness of the need to avoid stepping over the boundaries into the practice of medicine. My concept of myself as an independent nurse practitioner, embryonic as it was in the early days, had developed to the point where I knew how my knowledge and experience were to be used. Indeed, I could not in good conscience have hung out my shingle without a clear idea of what I could and could not do. I knew that the goal toward which medicine moves in applying knowledge and experience and the goal toward which nursing moves are different.

chapter four

Client contact— starting where the client is*

Of the utmost importance in professional nursing, as I have noted in previous chapters, is the art of truly "hearing" what the person seeking nursing care is expressing. It is this expression of the client's needs that will design the course of the professional nursing to be given. When I started my practice, therefore, I would carefully record what a client was telling me, writing on a tablet balanced on my lap. As I have also previously commented, I never met with a client with the physical and psychological barrier of a desk between us. Instead, the client and I sat just as visitors in a living room would sit. And I would listen. The notes taken at that first encounter with a client would become the client's health history, and as my practice evolved, the process of taking the health history became increasingly refined.

* This chapter had originally been titled "Health History Technique." It was changed to "Client Contact—Starting Where the Client Is" as a result of the question of a professional nurse at Milwaukee County General Hospital—Kathleen Hanson. Her question was, "History connotes the past, getting information about the past. You stress the importance of starting where the client is. Why do you call it a 'health history'?"

At first there were several caveats in the back of my mind. I was conscious, for example, of the possibility that physicians would claim that I was practicing medicine by taking a health history. I feared also that professional nurses would dismiss my practice as being something old, saying that they had always done precisely the same thing. In addition, I, myself, was struggling with the application of a concept, struggling not to lose it as I was giving nursing care. The result could have been a subtle slipping back into the old approach to a person, an approach that was secure and safe, but not truly professional. So in the early days, when I recorded what a client was telling me, I made marginal annotations that might serve as future rebuttals against any possible contention. As I listened to the client, I took upon myself the twin burdens of taking an accurate health history and of defending the act of taking that history. I knew also, of course, that the essence of professional care lay in the reasoning I engaged in as I moved toward making a nursing judgment, so a detailed account of that mental process as part of a complete health history was indeed vital.

Because of the vagaries of the process of recall, I wrote carefully, avoiding abbreviations, and I tried to record all that the person was saying to me and that I said to him. However, the distractions described above as caveats were evident in the way I initially recorded the health history and in the mental set that I had. When did this reticence leave me? I cannot pinpoint the exact time, but as I gave nursing care day by day, my focus shifted. Soon the real purpose of taking a health history surfaced to a conscious level. That is, I began to realize that as I let the clients speak freely, they were indeed telling me about *themselves* in a unique way, which was not limited to a specific "problem" or "condition" heretofore identified. Instead, what they expressed represented a composite, which might include aspects of a "problem" or "condition," but which, importantly, included other aspects of their lives seen by them as constituting a significant need. It was a need that could be expressed only in a health context that did not structure—and hence limit—the expression and identification of the need. There was a subtle difference entering my perceptions of the clients and their view of their needs. Of course, this subtlety was the core of the difference between what the person focused on when he went to see a physician and when he went to see a professional nurse. Although the difference was in my mind, I had not been able to verbalize it satisfactorily. There is a discomfort associated with knowing something as an idea and not finding the language to express it. I was emerging from a kind of intellectual hibernation. Over the years, layer after layer of frustrated searching had covered the essence of what I am now practicing and articulating. As my practice unfolded, these layers sloughed off, and what took their place was a sense of wonder and excitement, as there evolved between us—client and nurse— a concrete expression of this new relationship between a professional nurse and a person seeking her care. The relationship is portrayed in the phases of the health history that I have identified and that I will describe in this chapter. The health history, by the way, is more and more emerging in my mind as a tool that should be called a "nursing history."

The first and perhaps most important difference between the history that I take from a nursing perspective and that which is taken from a medical perspective is that in nursing, the relating of information is not really a history per se. I mean that what has previously happened to, for or with the person is not nearly as important as where the client is now in regard to the past. Whereas in medicine it is impossible to make an accurate diagnosis without a careful history of the patient's past medical events, it is possible to give nursing care without knowledge of the past. Hence the consummate importance of letting the client lead the nurse (as opposed to the nurse leading the client), of starting where the client *is* (as opposed to where the professional person feels he *ought to be*). The client will communicate to the nurse the points that are important to him, and in the initial stages this is all that the nurse should work with. Nursing care can definitely be given when the client tells where he is now. For example, the client who, in relation to either physical or mental pathology, says to me—"I have been through hell. I have been able to pull myself out of the depths with the help of medical personnel, and now I want to stay healthy, to hold on to the progress I have made. I know myself well now, and I can avoid certain things that would be dangerous to my continued health. Keep me from going back." Here I do not touch the past. Only that which my client tells me about the past as I am giving him care in the present do I incorporate into my nursing therapy. Another example is the client who said to me on the first appointment, "Can I start on the day of my accident? I was shot on the left side of my abdomen." To this day I do not know the circumstances of the actual shooting. I know who shot her, where she received medical treatment, that the bullet is still in her body. (I have palpated it.) But only as my client unfolds parts of the episode do I concern myself with that background.

The approach of letting the client move at his own pace has enabled him to handle favorable and unfavorable points about himself in relation to his needs in a very constructive way as he is helped by me in the exercise of his self-care agency. When the client introduces a medical aspect of his state of health, I place the information in the context of nursing, so that the medical history is part of the nursing history:

> Client recounts his health history and expresses his needs, disclosing his understanding and concerns about many aspects of living. Medical aspects may be expressed by the client as he sees his need. If the client does not mention medical aspects, they should *not* be introduced by the nurse.

In contrast to this approach, which is free-flowing, at the pace of the client, the medical history is a structured device, largely in question and answer form, designed to elicit information from the patient so that a set of signs and symptoms can be systematically identified and thus lead to an accurate diagnosis of disease.

As the purpose of the health history rose to a conscious level, the history indeed became a tool to help me give nursing care. At that point the old nursing frame of reference was abandoned, along with anxiety about projected comments from colleagues, which became a secondary concern.

Initially, as I had listened to my client, my mind had been clouded by this orientation:

1. Be sure to show why it is not medicine.

2. Be sure to show why it is nursing.

3. Be sure to show the effectiveness of my nursing care.

About one and a half years after the start of my practice, my mental set changed to:

1. The client is talking—LISTEN.

2. What he is saying to me and what I am saying to him become the manifest of nursing care. The health history is one of the tools I use to give nursing care.

About two years after the start of my practice, I was able to identify phases in taking the health history. The development of these phases was the result of my giving nursing care to a succession of clients. In 1971 I had only the most general idea of what would happen between me and my clients. The newness of the setting and the changed concept of nursing introduced a new element—the uncharted, unpredictable voicing of need by the client.

Medical History *Patient*	*Nursing History* *Client*
1. Nature of history known	1. Nature of history not known
2. Judgments about the history are predictable	2. Judgments about history are not predictable
3. Courses of action are identified	3. Courses of action are not identified

As I continued in my practice, I began to discern the unfolding of a pattern, and impressions began to crystallize about the effectiveness of my approach, often verified by my clients. To analyze the flow of the contact between my client and me, I reflected on what I had done from the moment of greeting the individual as he entered my office. I discovered that a truly therapeutic type of nursing care begins at that very moment. This is unique to the profession of nursing. Therapeutic nursing care must be given to the person from the instant of contact, and

must continue to be given as the client unfolds his reason for
seeking nursing care. I have not yet fully captured a description
of this type of nursing, but I predict that after it has been identified, it will one day constitute a segment of the courses in nursing education. The judgment about which kinds of nonverbal
and verbal communication to use at this point is so vital to the
continuation of effective nursing care that the importance of the
process can be equated with the extremely careful choice of the
point of impact used when dividing a diamond.

Although a clear description of moment-of-
contact nursing cannot yet be objectively described, I can offer
a subjective appraisal based on what clients have expressed to
me. To summarize the observation of one client—there is an
element of nursing care intrinsic to the practice of nursing in an
independent setting. As detailed in a previous chapter, heretofore a person in a medical setting could express health concerns
only as they related to the identification of a particular disease
and only in response to specific questions asked by the nurse or
physician when the medical history was taken. In that way, the
client's expression of needs was structured to follow a prescribed
path leading to a predetermined end—diagnosis and treatment
of disease. However, the nursing client perceives that he is receiving nursing care as a function of the mere availability of a
health professional in a setting in which he, the client, has the
freedom to express fully his health concerns, to request information, etc. (without feeling the pressure of "taking up the doctor's time"; without feeling the embarrassment of being cut off
when the nurse or physician considers his comments extraneous
to the immediate medical matter at hand; or without feeling the
frustration of receiving a patronizing reply or general comment
such as "It's nothing to worry about," which summarily dismisses
the person's concern, but leaves him nonetheless frustrated and
unenlightened). Thus, when a health professional in nursing
presents herself in a setting that encourages free expansion, in
which there is no pressure of time or of tradition, nursing care
is received as the client's expression of needs is facilitated, and
as the release results in a decrease of anxiety or frustration on
the part of the client. "There is something inherently thera-

peutic," my client said, "in just being able to talk with a professional nurse who listens to your concerns and helps you put them into perspective with regard to your health."

In my practice, as I began to focus fully on the client in my presence, the phrase in the nursing literature, "Start where the person is," (the word "patient" is traditionally used) began to take on new dimensions. As my mental set shifted to this concentration on what the client was saying, I became aware of my conscious effort *not* to make a judgment in tandem with the person's remarks, *not* to come up with an instant analysis or a conclusion about the significance of what he was saying at that particular moment, even if his remarks seemingly had all the classic characteristics of the feelings of, for example, guilt, depression or anxiety. It was a struggle for me to refrain from moving to reassure the client during the communication process, to refrain from preempting his next comment with a "yes, I know-what-you-mean" kind of statement. The pitfall of making premature judgments—which will lead to invalid conclusions, which will lead to poor judgments, which will lead to ineffective nursing therapy—cannot be overemphasized.

I would like to single out the use of process recording in the traditional settings with respect to the preceding sentence. In a process recording, the interpretation by the nurse of what the patient is saying is made during a brief contact with the patient. Subsequently, a conclusion based on the interpretation is recorded on the chart. Because of the brevity of contact and the possibility of superficial judgments, this is a very hazardous activity. Sometimes the conclusion is accurate; many times it is erroneous. In my practice, in trying to determine exactly where the client was, I became aware of a component of listening that I had not heretofore experienced. Full listening demanded that I erase everything from my mind, effecting a true *tabula rasa*. Then, and only then, did I really absorb what my client was saying to me. In the early days of my practice it took a concerted effort to erase everything from my mind, in view of the reservations I initially experienced.

In 1973, I identified five phases in the taking

of a health history at the time of the initial contact with the client, and in 1976 I added a sixth phase.

Phase   I—Greeting of the client by nurse

Phase   II—Client is speaker; nurse is listener

Phase III—Clarification of history by nurse

Phase IV—Judgment in regard to self-care assets and deficits

Phase   V—Establishment of a therapeutic self-care demand; goal-setting with client

Phase VI—Prescription of nursing therapeutic measures in light of assessed exercise of self-care agency

Taking the history involves a number of elements that are crucial to nursing effectiveness throughout the six phases, although they may vary in degree of implementation in each phase. They are:

1.   Waiting for client to express himself

2.   Timing of words in nursing response

3.   Tone of voice of the nurse

4.   Facial expression

5.   Precision of words

6.   Showing reactions

7.   Accepting the person where he is and accepting what his goals are at that time

Each phase will be discussed in the order of its occurrence. The following diagram is an outline of the phases identified from my practice in a five year period. These phases are those related to the initial client contact of approximately one hour's duration.

INITIAL CLIENT CONTACT
Time: Approximately one hour

PHASE I

CLIENT	greeted by	NURSE
Posture assumed, facial expression, and verbal expression		Notes these points

PHASE II

CLIENT	NURSE
Talks and is not interrupted. He is given time for full scope, emphasis and even repetition	Listens and records verbatim, maintaining eye contact with client

PHASE III

CLIENT	NURSE
Listens	Speaks—but only for clarification of recorded notes, such as something not clearly heard, unclear dates, etc. Tone of voice is important

PHASE IV

CLIENT	NURSE
Listener primarily	Speaker primarily Offers valid comments about self-care assets and deficits Timing is important Tone of voice is important

PHASE V

CLIENT		NURSE
Speaker primarily	←—————————→ Identification of therapeutic self-care demand; goal setting	Listener primarily

PHASE VI

CLIENT	NURSE
Listener primarily	Speaker primarily Prescribes nursing measures in light of therapeutic self-care demand

In the following pages, the phases will be discussed in detail in terms of the nursing care that is given in each one.

A discussion of the phases during which the knowledge base of the nurse is active and the phases during which judgments must be made in regard to what the client has said is very important. The following diagram illustrates that the use of the nurse's knowledge is appropriate in every phase of the client contact. However, the time at which she makes judgments is restricted. *It is extremely important to refrain from making premature judgments.*

PHASES	In the Nurse's Mind
I Greeting the client	No judgments made; knowledge base active
II Narration by client	No judgments made; knowledge base active
III Clarification by nurse	No judgments made; knowledge base active
IV Self-care assets and deficits	Judgment made; knowledge base active
V Therapeutic self-care demand	Judgment made; knowledge base active
VI Prescription of nursing measures	Judgment made; knowledge base active

Although the nurse's knowledge base is active throughout the entire contact with the client, a winnowing process must be engaged in, the client himself being the criterion for the selection of the material from the total fund of knowledge. In Phases I, II, and III it can be seen that no judgments are made. However, after sufficient evidence has been gathered from the client and understanding of the material is verified, then the nurse must make judgments. This process is noted as taking place in Phases IV, V, and VI.

PHASE I Greeting the client

A contrast must be drawn here. In traditional settings, it is difficult for a nurse to greet a person without overtones of a social situation. Other professions permit a small degree of crisp efficiency when their members come in contact with the individual. But it has become routine for nurses in the traditional setting to ask the person about his comfort, comment on the weather, be pleasant, fill the silence with conversation, etc. Indeed, observance of the social amenities—"being nice"—has often been confused with a *nursing* approach. The nurse's desire to help people, coupled with observance of the social graces, has conveyed to the public a mixed image of the function of a nurse.

In addition, the "continuing" aspect of nursing, divided into eight-hour periods, does not promote the notion of a ratio of economy of time to the service rendered. For example, it is unusual for an individual to receive one hour of professional nursing care per day in traditional settings because of the nature of his needs, and yet the ratio of professional nursing hours to patients is very high. On a "slow day" the continuing presence of the professional nurse sometimes leads to "chatting" with the patients. It explains, in part, the difficulty of having patients who expect to be "waited on" and the backlash effect of that expectation—seen when professional nurses abandon the patients to fend for themselves, offering as a reason the benefit of a speedier recovery if the person does things for himself.

In greeting my clients, I refrained from any small talk. I was direct and warm in my approach. I asked them to sit down either in a chair or on the small sofa in my office. As my practice grew, I became aware of the increasing difficulty of meeting the demand to blot out all distractions, all thought processes about other commitments, all reactions in regard to decisions in the making, of whatever magnitude, that had occupied my full attention just a few moments previously. This was especially difficult because I had no secretary to handle necessary paperwork, and my full-time teaching responsibilities, plus an increasing number of invitations to speak at various functions, demanded control and cataloging of many details in my life. This restriction of thought, of course, is the complete opposite of what I had been taught in the traditional settings, where I was told that a good nurse would be able to juggle simultaneously many separate pieces of knowledge and act on all of them.

In 1973 the practice was growing, I was still teaching, and in my personal life I was concerned about my elderly father. If a phone call, other communication, or even a thought came to my attention five minutes before a client appointment, I had to quell deliberately any further considerations related to the subject. Often this meant mentally closing the door and risking the loss of three or four vital details of matters that were on my mind, such as following through on a request, or persevering with busy telephone signals and lunch hours in attempts to contact someone. When my office door opened and

I saw the client, it was imperative that I fully and totally concentrate on him, absorbing every wave of communication emanating from him. Again, from a research point of view—to assure the purity of the data collected—I had to establish a setting free of possible contaminating influences. For the two valid reasons of good care and sound research, it was imperative that I be mentally decontaminated and thus render the setting sterile of variables, with only my client and me as subjects for analysis in structuring the body of nursing knowledge. "Getting down to business" in a nursing situation is different from "getting down to business" in a lawyer's or in a physician's office because a type of nursing therapy starts immediately in nursing, whereas there is delay in the other two instances. The lawyer has to hear an outline of the facts of the case before he initiates legal action on behalf of his client, and the physician has to hear the signs and symptoms before he initiates medical therapy. I believe that the immediacy and continuity of the therapeutic aspect of care given in nursing is intrinsic to the nature of nursing and that this can serve to delineate nursing action when other actions exist in a given situation. Phases of legal action and medical therapy can be administered in the absence of the client and patient through someone else—in the case of the lawyer, messages regarding court dates, obtaining necessary papers, etc.; and in the case of the physician, ordering medication and giving injections. Therapeutic nursing care cannot be given in the absence of the client.

As so often happens in life, a departure from routine because of necessity or extenuating circumstances often unfolds as an improvement or as an intrinsic part of the action attempted. Had I set up my office in the traditional way, with a receptionist with whom clients would check in, I would have missed the significance of the nursing care that is given by personally greeting the client. (Note: When I designed the space for my branch office in Bowie, Md., I put the secretary's office back of my office, so that when a client came in, I would be the one to greet him. This arrangement surprised the contractor who was helping me with my plans.)

In terms of nursing care, this arrangement does provide a client with continuity in contact and communication. That is, presumably when a person enters the office he has something on his mind, a concern that has motivated him to seek the services of a professional nurse. In my arrangement, his expression of needs is not fragmented among various office workers or assistants. A client has offered this example to contrast with the arrangement in my office: Upon a first visit to a physician's office, a patient usually checks in at the front desk and is asked to fill out a form. The form usually asks the patient to give in a few words the reason for the visit. Already, of course, the patient's expression is being structured. Once the patient is inside the physician's examining room, a nurse may take a medical history, during which the patient is asked to answer specific questions. He may feel the desire to begin to express his health concerns more fully. But his expression is guided by the specific blanks which must be filled in by the nurse. By the time the person sees the physician, he may twice have begun to "open up" about his health concern, but he may twice have been restricted by office procedure. In addition, the demeanor of the first two persons the patient encounters in the office—for example, the courtesy of the receptionist, or the manner in which the nurse elicits responses from him—will undoubtedly affect his ability to express his concerns fully when he reaches the physician's office. He may then place restrictions on himself, according to the cues he has received in the first two stages of his office visit. By the time the physician sees a patient, variables of which he is unaware may already have worked to restrict the communication forthcoming from his patient. And as the physician reads the forms filled out by the patient and nurse, his view of the patient is structured accordingly. Such a procedure in the medical setting may not necessarily decrease the efficiency demanded, since it is presumed that the physician will do his best to search out all the possible signs and symptoms so that he can accurately reach a diagnosis. However, in nursing, in which the emergence of needs results from the client's uninhibited communication, it is especially important that no such variables precede contact with a client. Whatever concerns were on his mind when he entered the office would not be sidetracked or buried, I decided, in setting up my office. I would not let office procedure be the antecedent to my nursing care.

In explanation of the diagram at the beginning of this chapter, I would like to note first that the verbal greetings I give my clients have continued to validate the importance I attached to the initial contact with the clients. In the early days there was a degree of mild uneasiness, or uncertainty, about "what to do." Fairly well established patterns exist in regard to keeping an appointment with the dentist, physician or lawyer. For my clients, it was different to be greeted by the professional person—the nurse—and not by a receptionist. It was different not being told, albeit in the form of a request, what to do: e.g., "Mr. X, how are you today? Have a seat. Dr. Y will see you shortly." Then, later, "Mr. X, will you come back to the first room on the left? Take off your jacket and shoes and unbutton your shirt. You can sit on the side of the table until Dr. Y comes in." So, when my client came in, and I greeted him and stayed with him, asking him to make himself comfortable, it was a new experience for him. The comment he made was usually consistent with my observation of his posture, his facial expression and his behavior. These observations were important because they supplied facts to be considered along with other aspects of himself that the client presented in regard to his needs. These observations, because they constituted data on which judgments would be made subsequently, had to be recorded and viewed as objective findings in Phase IV, when my judgment had to be incorporated into the client's perspective of his need. Some day, by means of video tape, I would like to help the person see what I see when he comes in, so that additional validation can be provided.

PHASE II   Client speaker, nurse listener

After I had invited the client to be seated and he had chosen a place to sit, I would open my spiral notebook and ask the client how he would like to be addressed. Then I would explain the nursing concept within which I would be recording what he told me. I would generally explain the process to the client in this way—or in simpler terms, when appropriate:

I shall be listening to everything you say and taking it down as you say it, because what you say is very important. I shall then look at what you say in light of the concept of my nursing care, which focuses on self-care assets and deficits, and from these, I will arrive at my nursing diagnosis of therapeutic self-care demand. Deficits, by the way, do not imply any deficiency on your part; they are what you need help with in overcoming or changing or initiating a health practice. I will focus on the exercise of your self-care agency. From time to time, I will share with you my judgments as the appointment progresses, and then I shall suggest some nursing care measures which I think will be of help to you.

None of my clients ever expressed confusion, incredulity, skepticism, dismay or rejection after such an explanation. They would respond with something like "Fine," and without further hesitation begin their own narrative. Sometimes I would have included in my explanation the observation that this would not be similar to a physician's medical history; and it soon became obvious to me that they had not expected it to be like one. Some would ask, however, "Are you going to ask me questions?" or, "Where do you want me to begin—what do you want to know?" or, "I suppose you want to know my medical history?" My response to these questions was a half-nod, a smile and usually the comment, "Wherever you would like to begin would be fine." The client would usually pause and then decide whether or not he wanted to include the medical aspects. If the medical aspects of the client's health state were important to him, he would tell me. If they were not important to him at that point, I did not make them important by asking questions about his medical past, thus directing his train of thought about his health concerns. If he talked about the medical aspects, it usually was necessary for me to make observations and ask some questions to obtain a complete picture of the medical aspects introduced by the client.

The cue to start the history comes from the client, and with one or two exceptions, all of the clients began immediately to express their concerns. One of these exceptions was a nineteen-year-old man who knew that his mother was (and is) a client of mine. He had initiated the idea of an appointment with me and told his mother of his intention. After I greeted him and oriented him to my nursing approach, he fell into an uneasy silence. I perceived the natural reticence of a nineteen-year-old and judged that nursing care was needed to put him more at ease. I applied some principles of psychology of the teenager. I find that an adult is more comfortable initiating the interaction and focusing on himself and his needs. However, the pressure on a teenager is great when he must focus concentrated attention on himself in the presence of another. For that reason, I initiate the conversation with a teenaged person. In this instance, I sensed that a need for a marked degree of privacy was an outstanding trait of the individual. I made a nursing judgment and followed through on it with the nursing measure of asking him how he wanted to be addressed, thus deliberately not assuming a degree of intimacy. "Shall I call you Mr. ———, or Tom, or Tommy?" I asked. "Tommy will be fine," he replied with a smile. I wrote that response in my book, forming the letters a bit more slowly than usual. He was still quiet when I looked up at him and smiled. So I continued. "You know," I said slowly, "I make a point of asking how my clients like to be addressed because it is my view that in today's society sometimes people intrude on each other's privacy." I observed him carefully as I spoke in measured tones and words. His face relaxed, then it took on a degree of intensity in the effort to hear what I was saying. "For example," I continued, "on initial contact one person will call another by his first name without asking permission and even worse will ignore the last name completely. This, of course, involves a loss of identity to a degree; concern about identity is evidenced by the way teenagers refer to Betty—whose mother plays the organ at church—or Jim—whose father owns the garage—in an effort to separate all the Bettys and Jims. Conforming to mores to a moderate degree is a sign of security and of a sense of one's identity; a marked degree can be a sign of insecurity and of loss of one's sense of identity. . . ." At this point, Tommy spoke. "I hadn't thought about it like that before, and that may explain my reason for being here better than I could have explained it. You see, my palms are terribly sweaty and I'm overly conscious of it. And I don't like people to come up and be aggressive in greeting—like, 'Hi, are you Tommy?' or 'What's your name?' 'Tommy?' 'Hi, Tommy!' I like to get to know people more slowly. I thought something was wrong with me."

    As I listen to a client, I write and simultaneously keep eye contact with him. This surprises the client at first, but soon he is unmindful of the movement of my hand, as indeed I am, myself. Practice through repetition honed my skill in doing all three things simultaneously—listening, writing and retaining eye contact. During Phase II, I noted the essentiality of my not speaking, even when the client fell silent for a period. *Intense listening proved helpful to the clients.* In the early years, I was not sure when the client had completed his account of his needs, or whether or not he was debating how to phrase the next point. Sometimes, he thought he was finished and would then recall something else. And I realized that premature speech on my part would have blocked additional information in several instances. I had to devise a way to be certain that my client had indeed finished and was ready to hear any comments I might make in light of what he had told me. On the other hand, I could not seem to the client to be unaware that he had finished. So, I found myself marking time in one-second beats, and a period of eight seconds seemed an appropriate length of time to wait. Next, I chose a gesture of eight-seconds' duration that would convey impending change in the speaker-listener roles. The gesture consisted of wetting my lips slowly with my tongue, turning back one or two pages of my notebook, taking a short breath with my laps parted and . . . if at that point the client added nothing else, I would speak. However, if he hadn't finished, the gesture gave him a clue that I perceived the lull as a termination point and provided him with a subtle nudge to continue. On occasion, at that point, the client would say, "Oh, yes, one more thing. . . ." I would start writing again, confident that I had not harmed the flow of communication. When it seemed appropriate again, I would employ the eight-second technique anew, until the client had truly reached a termination point in his communication to me. Then, we would continue into the next phase.

In the "Client speaker, Nurse listener" phase, no judgment is exercised in relation to the need of the client. The absorption in what the client is saying cannot be over-emphasized. In the diagram at the beginning of the chapter, you will note that the nurse is saying nothing. The client is speaking and the nurse is listening with every faculty of her being. The client is speaking, and whatever he says is significant.

PHASE III   Clarification

In this phase, the client became the listener and I became the speaker—the mental gears had been given time to shift. Since silence on my part was so essential in Phase II, I could not at that time clarify some points of the health history content. Let me establish the importance of distinguishing between clarification and verification. In Phase III, the clarification process consists in making certain that the nurse has a clear idea of the sequence of events, of family relationships, of locations of events, of dates, etc. If the nurse is operating under the impression that an individual mentioned by the client is his brother, for example, when in reality the person is his uncle, the direction the nurse takes in establishing nursing measures may be skewed from the direction in which the client is moving as he hears the words of the nurse. The effort to establish absolute clarity in regard *only to what the client has disclosed to the nurse in Phase II* assures better understanding in the subsequent interaction. Also, it is important to note that clarification does not include probing. And there should be no nursing judgments rendered in this phase.

The diagram on page 58 shows that there is an exchange between the nurse and the client. The nurse takes the initiative, since it is necessary for her to be completely certain of clarity in regard to what the client has said. In the next phase she exercises her judgment about his nursing needs, and it is a hindrance to nursing care if the nurse is using a point of departure that has incorporated into it some inaccurate understanding of what the person has said. It is important for the nurse to guard against letting clarification slip into verification of her growing notion of what the client's need is. That is one of the reasons why the tone of voice of the nurse is so important in this phase. A deliberately measured speaking pace is effective in this phase, and will help the nurse achieve an inquiring tone of voice.

PHASE IV   Judgment in regard to self-care assets and deficits

In the fourth phase, I began to form judgments about the self-care assets and the self-care deficits of my client. The technique that is all-important in this phase is one of slowness, deliberateness and precision. I wanted my client to be aware that I was bringing to bear all of my knowledge and experience in making statements about him and his self-care assets and deficits, that I was applying my whole being to helping him. The precise choice of words is extremely important, as are the tone of voice and the mannerisms that accompany the words. The client's expression of need dictates the choice of words in each instance. A study of detailed nursing cases is necessary to illustrate suggested approaches in the use of words appropriate to the need. However, the following episode provides an example of the kind of nursing care that can be categorized according to predictive manner of speaking, tone of voice, and choice of words:

One of my clients has been diagnosed as having Altzheimer's disease, and is in a nursing home. In this disease, the organic destruction of brain cells produces in the individual total inability to concentrate on anything for more than five or ten seconds and a heightened awareness of and sensitivity to noise, other activity, and the pressures of prodding. Chatter and cajoling, as techniques of persuasion, are contraindicated in nursing an individual with this disease. Yet I have observed a professional nurse approach the individual with a bright, loud greeting and ask him about a group activity in which he had been involved the previous day. This occurred immediately after I had succeeded—using a quiet, carefully measured manner of speaking—in having him sit down and remain relatively calm. Cajoling as a technique, often termed "persuasion," can sometimes be detrimental in the care of individuals, especially older persons who sense a tone of tolerance usually reserved for use with children. This behavior on the part of the nurse usually conveys undertones of arrogance and control to the older person, whose resulting reaction and resistance may be an attempt to verbalize: I am a grown person. I have a unique dignity that only age can bestow on a human being.

I can offer another example in which the manner of speaking must be appropriate to the situation. One of my clients is an 81-year-old woman. Her sister, aged 79, called me and made an appointment for a house call to conduct a physical examination of the woman because, she said, "She doesn't seem to be feeling well and I'm worried." After I had completed the physical examination, which showed findings within a normal range, I addressed myself to her state of personal hygiene. Her sister related that her efforts to bathe the woman, cut her toenails and fingernails (which were 1¼ inches long), comb her hair, etc. had been fruitless and had been met with hostility and anger. I drew up a chair facing the woman and said as simply and clearly as I could, using even tones, "I would like to make you more comfortable." A pause of five or six seconds followed. "Doing what?" she asked. "I would like to cut your fingernails." There was a pause. "No, they're all right," she replied. I nodded. "Fine." Her sister said, "See? Isn't it awful?" About two minutes later, I repeated everything exactly as before, with the same results. The third time, after an interval, I repeated my original words and added, as I gently took her hand, "See, they need cutting." She looked at her nails, and did not say anything. After another interval, I said, "Will you let me cut your nails? They need cutting. I think you will be more comfortable." This time, she looked at her hands and nails, held them out to me, and said, "They do need cutting." After I finished cutting her fingernails, I said, "Next time, I'll soak your feet and cut your toenails." On the next house call, I soaked the woman's feet and cut her toenails, and the next time I gave her a bed bath. Now she is beginning to dry herself, she takes off and puts on her clothes, is wearing shoes, and, according to her sister, her hearing is much improved.

The difference between the effectiveness of the nurse and the failure of the sister in accomplishing such measures lies mainly in the time given to the older sister to re-linquish her control of the situation. There is a subtle pressuring that a family member applies when a relative resists; this, in turn, causes some anxiety on the part of the one resisting and causes her to intensify her stand. In general, there is a prevail-ing lack of trust in relatives when they are being cared for by a member of the family. Perhaps they fear that the change they know has taken place in themselves will cause them to be re-jected by the family. When their needs exceed the family's abil-ity to care for them, they are removed from all that is familiar, and indeed, in the mind of the incapacitated individual, his lack of trust is justified and then he begins to distrust and fear every-one. In this particular instance, my voice carried a different message to the older sister, and yet she was with her family, which made her feel secure.

In law and other professions, the professional can and probably should be direct, succinct, even abrupt in manner of speech about the client's needs, because the need is external to the client and can be analyzed in the light of the most objective of criteria—facts. Both lawyer and client view events. In nursing, the need is not external—indeed this is a need that touches the essence of self; both the client and professional nurse are viewing the client's thoughts, feelings, and physical state. The nurse is treading on sensitivities that can be described in their vulnerability and tenseness as the sensation conjured up in the phrase "hanging neurons and ragged dendrites." For this reason, the nurse must be *exquisitely delicate* in her touch, her tone of voice and "good taste." Muted voice levels are always appropriate, as are gentle, compassionate tones. The voice of the nurse is probably her most important tool, the use of touch being related to voice in its effectiveness. *Sincerity is a prerequisite to effecting nursing care through the use of voice and touch.*

In this phase, as the diagram indicates, the nurse, on the basis of facts, her experience, and the unique aspects of this client's needs, uses her judgment to reach the point of verbalization of the self-care assets and deficits of the client. Constantly she weighs the effect of her nursing care as she communicates to the client what she perceives as she exer-cises her judgment. Her voice should take on a more positive tone at this point, thus projecting support of the client.

The flow of identification of self-care assets and self-care deficits can be seen in the following example. The client referred to earlier (who had a bullet lodged in her back) expressed fear of damage to the kidney at the time of the entry of the bullet. She associated difficulty in emptying the bladder with the possible kidney trauma, but showed knowledge of the anatomy of the stomach and rejected the notion of the bullet being the cause of subsequent gastric disturbance.

Assets	*Deficits*
1. Knowledge of anatomy of stomach	1. Lack of knowledge about physiology of kidney and bladder in light of difficulty of urination
2. Spiritual strength	
3. Validity of decision in regard to medical therapy	2. Fear of having to go on kidney machine

The reader must be cautioned against drawing a conclusion about a medical condition—i.e., serious kidney disease—from the reading of these self-care assets and deficits. The client was concerned about a problem with urination. She feared that the gunshot wound had caused a cyst on her kidney (and would necessitate her having to go on a kidney machine), when in reality the cyst was unrelated to the wound. Continued nursing care is needed, however, to help her gain a perspective with regard to needed medical therapy.

It must also be underscored that the listing of these deficits in abbreviated form is but *a part* of the health history technique—hence the need to refrain from drawing conclusions prematurely.

PHASE V   Identification of therapeutic self-care demand

I entered the fifth phase of the health history when I gave my client my nursing diagnosis of a therapeutic self-care demand—if I could arrive at one at that time. Otherwise, I advised the client that I would have to analyze further what he had told me, in order to formulate a nursing diagnosis later. I would then offer nursing care measures to achieve a goal that had been identified with my client as a desirable one. Thus, the appointment would draw to a close, if through the health history the client's expressed needs had been met or would soon be met. If, after the history, a physical examination was needed, or if the client requested specific health information, those actions would follow. Sometimes those actions would be reserved for a subsequent appointment, depending on the desire expressed by the client. Together, the client and I arranged for another appointment. Usually the client expressed the need to have one before I suggested that another appointment was necessary.

One kind of need that does require comment at this point is the need of a client to have an injection for an allergy, as therapy prescribed by a physician. The initial history in this case is brief and usually takes only fifteen or twenty minutes because of the specificity of the need. However, during subsequent visits, the client usually broadens his scope of needs as I sit with him in the time following the injection. Accordingly, the health history technique as described above is utilized to deal with the broader needs being expressed by the client. Thus, there is not necessarily an end to the professional nursing once a specific, limited goal has been reached. The nursing cycle moves with the needs of the individual.

This phase represents the point at which the nurse makes a decision that will affect the choice of nursing care measures she will recommend to the client. As the diagram indicates, an exchange between the nurse and the client is necessary. The client, participating in his self-care and exercising his self-care agency, must be aware of what the therapeutic self-care demand will require in terms of his understanding and willingness to follow through on short-term goals—to accomplish a long-range goal or goals. A therapeutic self-care demand may be described as a continuation of the self-care assets and deficits identified and given as examples in the preceding phase. A typical therapeutic self-care demand might be phrased as follows: *Therapeutic self-care demand*—the need to monitor details of the client's urination process (the urge to void, actual voiding, time element related to voiding) to help get an accurate picture of the functioning of her urinary system, which will help to pinpoint whether medical care is necessary.

In the contact with my client, he is the activator. He is helped in making a decision in light of what he has told me and in light of my professional nursing judgment. He then receives continued support in implementing his decision about where he wants to be in his health state. I do not pressure him into choices he does not want to make or is not yet ready to make. Clients have told me that they hedge with the physician at times, but they do not with me. They are not hesitant about disclosing themselves and their various emotions to me; there are no expectations of behavior and reactions on my part. The way in which I record the information the client gives me is a free-flowing one, because it is too early to design a general format or record. And it will always be necessary to allow for the free flow of information from the client, in order to prevent a limitation on that communication. No general classifications have yet emerged. The needs of individuals are unique, so that at least a thousand client cases would have to be analyzed before the broadest categorization could begin. Even though a broad classification will be necessary in order to form a body of nursing knowledge, it must never predetermine the nurse's approach to a client. The individuality of each person is the inexhaustible source of challenge, which, paradoxically, taps the source of creativity within the professional nurse. It is possible to classify diseases in detail, but people can never be classified to the same extent. Appendicitis may be the same in a thousand people, but a thousand people with appendicitis will never be the same. The variables of the knowledge base, motivation, goals, understanding, ability and perspective of individuals offer an infinite number of combinations in regard to the predictive aspect of nursing needs. Thus, the demand on the nurse is unique: the immediacy of judgment to be made; the resulting action that meshes a set of gears within the client—which necessitates another judgment on the part of the nurse—and so on in a continuing process. Therefore, the structured body of nursing knowledge is the point of departure, a rule of thumb, for the student of nursing as she begins her professional career. However, she must never mistake the body of knowledge for the process of nursing itself. For in preoccupying her mind with the general lessons of previous nursing, she may close her mind to the communication of needs currently emanating from her client, who is in totality like no other person in the world. And in this error she would lose the essence of professional nursing.

PHASE VI   Prescription of nursing therapeutic measures

I identified this phase in 1976. In analyzing the chronology of my awareness of it, I asked myself:

1. Was it there all the time, from 1971 on?

2. Had I interspersed the action, per se, through the other phases?

3. Why did it assume such definite shape only after the other phases had been clearly identified for a period of three years?

My analysis is this: The other five phases had to be perfected to the degree that I was able to discriminate between the significance of (1) the nursing judgment that supported self-care measures already taken by the client; (2) nursing judgments that more data needed to be gathered through application of certain measures; and (3) nursing judgments that were creative and original in selecting the combination of activities that would build on self-care assets and effect better health states in the clients. Obviously, this kind of judgment required a degree of self-confidence, of boldness, of risk of failure. In addition, I had been circumspect in the execution of the other phases, and this furnished me the necessary solid data from which I could proceed. I concluded that it was an evolutionary process and that therefore:

1. It was not there all the time through 1971–1976.

2. It had not interspersed the action, per se, through the other five phases.

3. A process of refinement, maturation and professional patina had to be acquired prior to acquiring the security of being creative.

My intellectual hibernation had ended.

chapter five

Physical
examination

When I started my independent practice, the
question of nurses giving physical examinations was not explored in the nursing literature to the extent that it is today in
nursing books and journals. For the most part, what did appear
in the literature dealt with the pediatric nurse practitioner and
her role in conducting physical examinations with a pediatri-
cian. In an effort to dilute the significance of what the nurse
would be doing, as compared to what the physician was doing,
the words "physical assessment" began to appear in the journals
—as if this designation somehow skirted the potential legal
problem of nurses performing such medical tasks. In the minds
of those who teach the technique of physical examination from
a medical perspective, the question was and is, How can the
line be drawn between making a primary medical diagnosis and
merely collecting information so that a physician can make a
medical diagnosis? I believe that the literature reflects a new
high in rationalizing the so-called expanded role of the nurse,
which includes the taking of medical histories and the performance of physical examinations. In reality, the inclusion of
these activities within the bailiwick of the nurse has expanded
not her nursing role per se, but her *medical* role. A more accurate description of the nurse's role in such situations is that

she is an extension of the physician, and what she is doing is, to a degree, practicing medicine at the most fundamental—and, it could be argued, the most critical—phase in the making of a medical diagnosis.

From the beginning of my practice, I knew that I should not approach a person with the idea of "zeroing in on a medical diagnosis." As I have indicated in previous chapters, I was aware of the hazard of presenting myself as a practitioner of medicine. And yet I had background knowledge of pathology that was called into play constantly as I functioned as an independent professional nurse. Here the premise mentioned earlier must be repeated: a nurse can know as much as or more than a physician, but the purposes to which this knowledge are applied can differ.

Gradually, I was able to articulate more precisely my concept of performing physical examinations and to describe the significance of doing an examination from a nursing perspective. Starting with the fact that the physical examination is a tool for gathering facts about a person, we know that the tool can be used by many professional people in many fields with different goals in mind. The goal, therefore, should be the focus in the use of the tool, and the tool itself should not be presumed to be useful for one purpose only. Once in the early days of my practice a physician asked me if I felt secure in making a diagnosis when doing a physical examination. "But I don't conduct an examination for that reason," I responded. "Oh, come on now," he said. "There's only one reason for doing a physical examination and that is to make a diagnosis." I answered, "In medicine, there may be only one reason, but in nursing, I do it for another reason. I do physical examinations to tell my clients what my eyes, ears and hands tell me about their bodies, so that I can help them make decisions about what they want to do in light of those findings." When I was able to phrase the difference in this way, I found myself becoming freer of any lingering doubts that I was somehow involved in the diagnosis of disease.

In addition, the techniques of palpation, percussion, inspection and auscultation are used by nurses many times throughout their careers. The idea of putting them all together in what is known as a physical examination, however, may cause the nurse to be reluctant to apply her knowledge, and she may feel that her knowledge is not commensurate with the purpose. In my practice, I approached the giving of physical examinations from the following perspective, as I crystallized the difference between the medical approach and my nursing approach:

PHYSICAL EXAMINATION

Nursing Reason	Medical Reason
To identify:	To identify:
What is right	What is wrong
How well the person is	How sick the person is
How healthy the person is	What disease the person has
Nursing Focus	Medical Focus
The person is the concern	The organ is the concern
Time given to person talking	Brief time is given
Self-care action	Passivity on part of patient
Starting where the client is in understanding	Starting with complaint and tests

With a reason and focus different from the traditional medical reason and focus, I was able to utilize all the knowledge I had acquired over the years. Even though my goal was learning about health, I began to feel the need to learn more about pathology—as an aid in helping my clients to understand their real or potential pathological states, so that I could design a nursing system based on their assets while considering their deficits. In my practice, I decided that the *question of the client,* expressed during the health history, would be the point of departure for me in handling the data I would obtain from the examination. I knew that I would communicate to the client what I perceived during the examination. Many times during my traditional nursing career I had told a patient what my ears heard, what my hands felt, and what my eyes saw. I decided I would use the same approach with my clients in my independent nursing practice.

Since I did not have the burden of making a medical diagnosis when conducting a complete or partial examination, I did not conduct a systemic exam. I set several criteria for myself, however. The first was comfort for my client, the second was a sequential pattern and the third was thoroughness of the total examination. I did not want my client to be inconvenienced by sitting down, sitting up, then lying down, turning over, sitting up again, etc. So I thought I would examine as much of the body as I could with the person sitting up. This would include examination of the head—eyes, ears, nose and mouth; and the neck—glands, arteries and veins. The chest would be examined anteriorly and posteriorly, and then the person would lie down and I would examine the chest again; then the abdomen and finally the extremities. A blood pressure reading was also included. If a pelvic examination was to be done, I would conduct it after completing the others, and I would draw the blood for tests after the examination. The usual tests are: complete blood count, glucose and cholesterol. Many clients request health profiles, such as an SMA 12. If, during the health history, the client manifested particular concern about one area—say a bunion on his foot—then I would first direct my attention to his foot, and then proceed with a sequence that would spare the client as much inconvenience as possible.

The growth and development of the individual being examined are important to consider. When I examine the head, I feel the contour of the skull, the looseness of the scalp, the intactness of the skin and the condition of the hair. The eyes should be bright and clear; the retinal wall orange in color and full; patent arteries and veins—red and blue-red, respectively. I look for open nasal passages with moist membranes. The mucous membrane of the mouth should be pink and very moist; the tongue smooth and pink, the pharyngeal area a deeper pink. The teeth should be white and intact in their structure as well as firm in their roots in the gums. The ears should be clear, with the cilia and a moderate amount of wax evident. The tympanic membrane should be glistening, pearly gray and intact. The skin of the face should be clear and pink and the texture firm. The neck should be straight and strong to hold the head high. The arteries should be felt for a strong, regular beat and the fullness of the veins observed. The glands and muscles of the neck are palpated for smoothness and the muscles for firmness and strength. The anterior and posterior chest are auscultated for the regular, rhythmic, clean beat of the heart and the sound of the air passing through the bronchi and the alveoli;

and the expansion of the chest on deep inspiration is measured. The abdomen is palpated and inspected for the position of the liver, spleen and kidneys, and the contents of the intestinal tract. The femoral arteries are palpated for a strong, regular beat. The extremities are inspected and palpated for the strength of the muscles and the warmth and intactness of the skin. The feet are inspected for contour, intact skin and warmth. The dorsalis pedis arteries are palpated for a strong regular beat. If a vaginal exam is done, the pink color, intact moist membrane and smooth cervix are noted. A smear of the secretions is taken to identify the normal cells.

During the course of the examination, attention is focused on normal, as opposed to abnormal, structure and functioning. I communicate to the client what I observe, hear, and feel. In addition, the client talks to me as the examination progresses, and thus I gain a perspective from the input of the client, as well as from what I ascertain objectively. *If pathology is present, it will almost always leap out at the professional nurse.* This point cannot be overemphasized, and the examples I shall cite will bear out this important realization. The results of the examination—the test findings and the data given by the client—invariably pinpoint the locus, nature and degree of possible pathology. The results are disclosed to the client and nursing care is directed toward assisting the client to choose a course of action in light of the results.

I have devised a way of assessing the health of the individual based on the findings of the physical exam. I evaluate the findings on a range of normal, using a scale of 1 to 10, such as this:

	Range of Normal										*Abnormal*
Head	1	2	3	4	5	6	7	8	9	10	10+
Neck	1	2	3	4	5	6	7	8	9	10	10+
Chest	1	2	3	4	5	6	7	8	9	10	10+
Abdomen	1	2	3	4	5	6	7	8	9	10	10+
Extremities	1	2	3	4	5	6	7	8	9	10	10+

The number 1 represents the most normal, and 10 represents the least normal. Anything over 10 becomes 10+ and falls within the range of abnormal findings. I make a judgment about where on the scale that person's findings seem to fall and then add up the five numbers to reach an overall picture of his positive health state. I do not identify a state of anatomy in my notes by the word "negative." The use of that word in medicine indicates the *absence of abnormality,* and in doing my physical examinations I want to tell my clients *what is present in terms of the normal.* The obvious result of this use of the words "negative" and "positive" is that the concepts conveyed by the findings are reversed. In my practice of nursing, a positive finding is desirable; whereas in medicine, a negative finding is desirable, in accordance with the medical purpose of a physical examination—to diagnose possible illness. To put it another way, in my practice of nursing, the use of the word "positive" conveys health to the client; in medicine the use of the word "positive" conveys illness. From the client's perspective, something that is positive is good for him, so a subtle change in viewpoint occurs, removing the impression that "positive" findings must have "negative" implications for his health. Some of my clients have even told others about me by saying, "She tells you what is positively good and right about you and your health state."

It is obvious that a reversal of approach must be effected by the professional nurse, who has been taught to know, evaluate and take action on the basis of disease, illness and pathology.

Let me take the point expressed earlier to illustrate the distinction I make in relation to use of the knowledge of a professional nurse and her application of it in doing a physical examination in the traditional setting. My comments about nursing on a general floor unit become more poignant when applied to nursing in intensive care units, coronary care units and trauma units and in other medically complex and medically fluid situations such as the emergency room. The facts are:

1. The nurse has come in contact with the patient because he has been admitted with a mental or physical condition that requires medical diagnosis and medical care. He is past the

time period of being at home, wondering, worrying and knowing that he will have to be treated medically.

2.   Subsequent observations on the part of the nurse are locked into the fact of illness.

3.   All the results of the nurse's inspection techniques, her auscultatory techniques and her palpatory and percussive techniques *must* relate to the fact of the medical condition, so that she can make early, astute and accurate observations *to the physician.* She must know, in a significantly circumspect way, the meaning of a change in the person from the pathological perspective. The burden and the pressure are great and give rise to these questions:

a) When is a knowledge of pathology sufficient?
b) Should not the nurse in this instance have knowledge commensurate with the physician's about the medical state of this particular patient? (If the answer is yes, the implications are clear.)
c) What criteria should be used in schools of nursing in selecting the content of courses about disease, as well as pathology?

Obviously, in my practice I do not have these pressures. Indeed, the approach is from the completely opposite perspective of helping the client to understand his concerns about his *health,* and thus to gather facts which he can use as a starting point in making his decision about seeking medical care when it is needed. Even using this approach, I do not negate the need for a knowledge of pathology and disease, *in depth*— and for the pursuit of ever-deepening knowledge. Because I record what is right, what is normal—e.g., the entire left lung has very good air exchange, and two lobes of the right lung have good air exchange—my client can start building on the positive findings. Contrast that with conveying to a client the information that the lower right lobe has something wrong with it, that there is interference with air passing through, that there is some fluid accumulating in the lung, etc. There is nothing in that last instance for the client to build on, to use as a strength. Through the use of the physical examination tool in my practice, the assets are communicated to the client along with the deficits, so that the building process involves preserving the assets and taking steps to turn the deficits into assets.

My new clients who hear me talk about a health assessment respond with comments that indicate a new view of themselves. One of my clients, who has a history of attempted suicide and has received treatment for various medical conditions, came to me because she was "tired all the time." When I spoke of doing an examination, including blood tests and an EKG, to get a health assessment—so that we could work with how healthy she is—she replied with delight, "*Health* assessment! What a marvelous idea! I hadn't thought of an examination that would tell me how well I am!"

The physical examination, like other aspects of my practice, emerged as a result of needs expressed by my clients. The first time I conducted a partial examination in my office was when a client, concerned about burning on urination, asked me to look at her urethra. At the time, I felt the uneasiness that accompanies most experiences occurring in a new setting. I had her prop her feet on a cocktail table—it was awkward—I dropped the flashlight—and I had difficulty making her comfortable. For subsequent clients, I put together two solidly constructed tables and padded them with blankets. The first complete physical examination I conducted on those tables went very well. Eventually, a colleague donated to my practice a padded table for physical examinations. But the important aspect of that era, during which the appropriate equipment was lacking, was that the need arose from the client. As I have previously mentioned, I had no prior idea of the needs the clients would present to me, and thus I did not prepare for the possibility of physical examinations. Also, I did not want to convey to my clients through the appearance of the office that I was offering substitute medical services. Literally, my physical examinations grew out of my clients' needs, their requests, and not out of my need to gather physical data. It was in effect a suggestion of the client, not of the professional practitioner, that led to the conducting of the physical examination and at the same time to the emergence of an important tool of nursing.

Of course, my self-confidence grew with each physical I conducted, and I soon lost the tension that I had felt at first. At this point I must identify a very important event in terms of my professional growth. It occurred in 1972, when Mrs. Roxanne Stigers, director of nursing at a nursing home, contacted me and asked me to give physical examinations to the employees of the home. Each was required to have an annual physical examination and was given the choice of being examined by a physician or by a professional nurse. The majority signed to have the examination done by me. That fact in itself was gratifying to me. Another significant fact was that the purpose of these examinations was consonant with the purpose of the examinations I conduct in my office. The purpose was to certify the health state of the employees, not to try to find something wrong with them. In addition, in a setting such as a nursing home, it is important not only for the employees to be free of obvious pathology, but also to be in the best possible state of health, in terms of sleep habits, adequate diet and exercise, etc., so that the home residents receive the kind of alert and patient (as opposed to impatient) attention that is needed. Thus, examinations and discussion with a professional nurse would afford the opportunity to focus on these positive health aspects. In addition, it is most unusual for a person not to seek a physician when he is feeling ill, so it could be presumed that if there had been a question of disease, the home employee would have chosen to see a physician. Even if there were something objectively wrong, which the person was unaware of, that fact would most likely be ascertained by an examination. In medicine, the signs and symptoms expressed by the patient provide important clues to the physician in making a diagnosis. Without such guidance, even medical science does not have all the knowledge necessary to discern pathology in its earliest forms in the human body, so even a physician cannot make a diagnosis in many instances until such symptoms are verbalized. There is, therefore, a fundamental error in the assumption that when pathology exists in a stage that can be observed, the nurse would not be able to see it just as the physician would. Thus, the examinations to verify the health states of employees of the home were natural ground for a professional nurse.

About 160 employees were to be examined. They included the home administrator, the director of nursing, professional and practical nurses, nursing aides, orderlies, volunteers, kitchen workers and janitors. Some family members of these individuals also came, and about ten continued with my care by making appointments to see me at my office. The examination that the nursing home and I had agreed on included: examination of the eyes, ears, nose, mouth, throat, neck, chest, vagina and extremities; blood pressure measurements and blood serology for syphilis. The employees indicated that they had never received such a detailed examination when they were working and healthy and when the physical was a routine one associated with their work.

When the employees came in for their appointments, they would make such comments as "I feel fine. You won't find anything wrong with me." They would hand me the two-page form listing possible medical conditions with the check marks in the "no" column. At that point, I would respond only by saying, "Fine!" I did not say, as I do now, "That's a good reason to come to me for a physical examination. I can help you identify what is keeping you well and help you to build on these points so that your chances of staying well will be greater." Perhaps my reticence was due to the fact that I had assumed responsibility for a large number of persons for the first time. Maybe it was in the back of my mind that I must not fail the nursing home by, for example, failing to pick up something that could harm the residents, such as poor personal hygiene after having a bowel movement or after taking care of an individual who was incontinent of feces. There was no place on the form for that kind of data. The clients would ask me questions about such things as diet, exercise, vitamins and birth control pills, and many times they talked with me about their marital problems or their worries about going to school while working. They seemed to sense that there was a difference between the physical examination that I gave and that given by their doctor. They would say, for instance, "I wanted to come to you because I knew I could talk to you about anything—it would not seem too small to bring up, and you would listen." After the physical examination, some would comment about the thoroughness of the exam as contrasted with a purely medical exam—"You have to be really sick to get that thorough an examination at a doctor's office!"

When I arranged with Mrs. Stigers to conduct the examinations, we discussed the time it would take for each examination. Among the several points considered were the facts that the examinations would be done on company time and that the employees would pay for the examination and laboratory tests, and the amount of time I felt could be given in proportion to the limited fee that would be charged. (Many of the employees had insurance coverage, so they would not have had to pay the full amount for an examination done in a physician's office.) After several days of doing the examinations, I noticed that the time for each was getting longer and longer, so I scheduled fewer appointments per day without increasing the cost to the employee. What was happening, of course, was that establishing the nurse/client relationship during each exam required a significant amount of time, because of the increased two-way communication involved; and this was increasing the length of each examination.

The whole experience, in short, was teaching me self-confidence—from a subjective point of view, because I could see progress in myself, and also from an objective point of view, because the evaluations written by the employees after the examinations were so favorable. In retrospect, at the time I had an uncomfortable feeling that what the employee clients and I had in mind regarding a physical examination was different from what the world of professionals traditionally expected a physical examination to be. *I was stressing the health of the individuals.* But the questions I heard from the professionals to whom I described the experience were along the lines of, "What was wrong with the *patients?*" and "How could you be sure you had not missed anything?" I would explain that it was not my purpose to reach a conclusion about the findings in terms of a diagnosis of a medical condition. The colleagues would look baffled and say, "Well, then, why would they come to you?" And I would respond, "Why should they come to me for a medical diagnosis? Why should I prepare myself to take on the responsibility of medicine and offer my services to the people as a more accessible, less expensive type of medical care—a kind that would make me vulnerable to the justified charge that I was practicing medicine? From the client's point of view, I would be offering second-rate medical care, and, most emphatically, that is not the kind of need that brought them to me. They do not expect that! Only the professionals seem to expect me to conduct that kind of an examination. And since I do not do that type of examination, but do approach the technique from the point of view of the client's need, I am making available to the client the kind of nursing care that he cannot receive in any other setting in our present health care system."

Perhaps the lack of understanding of why and how I conduct physical examinations and of what I do with the information gathered disclosed to me more than any other single factor the reality of the situation that in many minds—the minds of some professional colleagues and the minds of persons who are not my clients—a nurse performs medical acts in rendering care, but the physicians set the limits on what these acts are, on when they are carried out and on how they are carried out. I realized that I was coping with a concept alien to my own and that therefore others would not understand what I was trying to accomplish. I realized that most nurses do not see nursing as separate from medicine.

The following illustration will convey what I had discovered through my experience in conducting physical examinations and what had confirmed in my mind that my procedures were sound. I realized that the most important people—my clients—were in fact accepting my services and perceiving a difference between those services and what they would expect to receive from a physician. To the question "If you don't make a diagnosis when the person comes to you, and if you cannot prescribe medication, then why would anyone come to you?" I offer in reply the following diagram:

Person Who Has a Health Need

(Or who thinks he has one)

| I wonder? | I think. | I'm fairly certain. | I am sure. | What should I do? |

I have had clients come to me expressing their needs in these terms. Further, some clients said that if they had not had access to me, they would not have seen anyone about their health state. Another illustration helps to show the gap that exists in the delivery of health care services: Where can the person go with his questions and with his knowledge of himself and his health state?

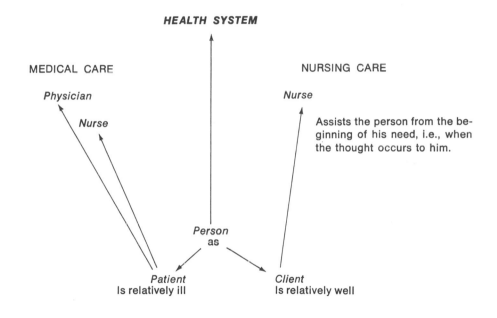

An example may clarify further this aspect of the health-illness continuum. When, for instance, a client identifies a change in himself that moves him closer to the illness side of the continuum, talking with a professional nurse affords a number of advantages. It puts into perspective what the client *himself* has noticed *about himself* and provides a professional judgment about the significance of it. From experience, I am able to identify pathology as opposed to nonpathology and in almost every instance the client, as he receives nursing care, gives the clue to which course of action he wishes to pursue. (Although sometimes the client is unaware that it is a clue, the professional nurse should detect it.) My clients have not indicated that they see me as a "screening step" in their health care; rather, they see my care with regard to the physical examination as clarifying and verifying information and as supporting them throughout. One can only reiterate here how inadequate a person can feel when faced with deciding whether he should see a physician on his own. In such a case, the nursing care process follows this sequence: Professional nursing care, first through the health history technique, helps the person to identify and express his health concerns and needs. Then, the physical examination tool transforms the process from what the client sees in himself to what the nurse sees in the client by means of the physical examination—armed as she is with the knowledge gained from the health history and from the client's comments during the physical examination. Putting together the information garnered from the health history and physical examination, the client and the professional nurse can view the health situation clearly, and the client is helped to make a decision. I have found, by the way, that given an understanding of the situation, people in general display good judgment about seeking appropriate care.

Involvement in the partial examination has always been part of the traditional routine of nursing; i.e., the nurse inspected (but it was called "observing"); she palpated (and it was called "feeling"); and she auscultated (and it was called "listening"). But the nurse's responsibility ended with making the proper notation on the chart, *so that the physician could then take action.* Now, however, using the same physical examination technique, but placing it in an *independent setting*, what does one do with the results? It is in this instance that the *professional* quality of what has been called professional nursing comes to the fore. Here the professional nurse exercises the crucial element of judgment—in putting the findings into perspective with the total health picture of the client; in helping the client to understand that health picture; and in helping the client to move to the point at which he can make a decision on a course of action in light of that health picture (a course of action that may include seeking medical care). In short, *the client, not the physician, takes action.* It can be clearly seen, then, that the focus of the nurse's information-gathering and judgment-making processes in the independent setting is the client. The goal is not to make the appropriate notations on a patient's chart, but to make the appropriate "notations" to *and with* a client. The end result may very well be that the client will seek medical care, and it may also be that the professional nurse will be asked by the client to communicate her findings to the physician to be consulted. The difference, of course, would be that her "findings" would be not isolated pieces of information, but an integrated picture of the client's health state, communicated along with the judgment of the professional nurse regarding that health state. Whereas in the traditional setting the construct would be:

patient (approached by) — *nurse* — (as an extension of) *physician*

The new construct becomes:

nurse (as extension of) — *client* — (who decides to seek) *physician*

In the independent setting, the client becomes the pivotal point.

I will illustrate my approach to physical examinations by giving examples of four clients whose nursing needs included either a partial or a complete physical examination at some point during my care of them. For the purposes of this chapter I have extracted from the records of total nursing care only those portions related to the physical examination. The uniqueness of the care lies in my determination of how to proceed, from the professional perspective of my practice, and how I used the tool of the physical exam.

One client came to me because she felt nervous, apprehensive and tense. She would try to relax but was not successful. She had just turned 50 years old and expressed self-depreciatory distress at the thought of growing old. "I have been to three physicians over the last two years and all of the tests have been negative. They tell me that my feelings are probably due to the menopause, to growing old, which I definitely don't like, and to the fact that my children will soon be leaving. In addition, the difficult years with an alcoholic husband have taken a lot out of me. But I still don't feel well, and I don't sleep well, and I'm just jittery all the time and everything gets on my nerves. I snap at people and get impatient and I don't like that trait in me. I just don't feel well, but all the tests are negative, so it must be in my head—it must be psychosomatic. So will you help me as to what to do now?"

Her health history was longer than that written above, but I have indicated the initial part, which explains her reason for seeking a professional nurse. I proceeded on the basis that three physicians had said nothing was wrong with her. I would have seen myself acting as a medical consultant had I said to her the equivalent of, "Well, let me do an examination with tests and let me see if I can find anything." In other words, I accepted what the client had said about the medical appraisal of her signs and symptoms and included the medical opinions in my approach to her nursing care. Part of my nursing care was to take into account her physiological state, and I established with her the need to keep a record of her physical feelings. "Even if your big toenail aches, if anything seems so minor you are tempted to disregard it, that's what you should write down," I suggested. She did keep a diary and said she found it helpful to her in several ways, one of which was that it allowed her to describe the frequency and degree of her "heart palpitations," her fatigue and her tension, and how well she slept at night. "I can't relax," she said. So I initiated exercises that would help her to attain a relaxed state. On her weekly visit, she would tell me that they helped quite a bit, at some times more than at others. She said she was feeling better, but the heart problems persisted. I had told her that if she experienced any of those feelings in my office to let me know immediately and I would stop and check them out. She had been coming to me on a weekly basis for two months and felt that her increased understanding of herself had contributed to her improved health state. One afternoon I was helping her carry out the relaxation exercises when she said, "There, there, there are those feelings. If I could draw a caricature of myself it would show me with a great big heart outside of my chest just pounding away ready to leap from my body." I said quietly, "Just stand there; don't move, and I'll examine you." I placed my stethoscope on her left carotid artery and heard a rapid but clear, clean pulse. I palpated the carotid artery and moved my stethoscope to the right carotid artery, with the same auditory results. I palpated the right carotid artery and then moved to palpate the glands in her neck. On palpation of the thyroid gland, I felt a nodule in the left lobe of the thyroid gland. I told her what I had heard and felt. As I have indicated, giving the client information about what I perceive is part of my concept of nursing. It is an integral part of the self-care regimen that a client understands his body and health state and thus can become an active participant in his self-care agency. In doing this, the professional nurse is not making a diagnosis, is not pinning a medical name on a condition, but is merely describing what she senses so that the client can act on the basis of that information. So I told her calmly and slowly, "You have a nodule on the left lobe of your thyroid gland." "I do?" she asked, with her hand at her side. "Yes," I said. "Feel it. Put your fingers here." She had difficulty feeling it and I told her to feel my thyroid and then to feel hers again. Finally she said, "Yes. I feel it. Yes, there it is." I suggested that we sit down and discuss what we had felt. She asked, "What do I do now?" In response, I suggested that she choose one of the four physicians she had seen previously and tell him what had been found. We then talked about thyroid scans and hot and cold nodules and the significance of each. We talked about possible medical and surgical therapies used in such situations. The client went to a physician and told him about the nodule. He advised surgery and asked which surgeon she wanted. She explained that she could not make that decision until tests had been done and until she had discussed it with her independent nurse practitioner. After the tests, which showed a cold nodule, she talked with me and decided to seek the opinion of another physician. At her request, I accompanied her when she went to see the new physician and stayed with her during her physical exam. After palpation, the physician said that he thought the nodule might be warm and that after tests he would recommend either medication or surgery. The second tests indicated a warm nodule, and my client then started on medication. Later, the nodule was much smaller and there were hopes that it might eventually disappear.

This client presented needs within the general categories of "I'm fairly certain" (something is wrong) and "What should I do?" In this case, professional nursing helped her to verify and clarify her feelings and to make a decision about a course of action; and then supported her throughout the chosen course.

Another example is a client who is in her late sixties. She came to me because she was not feeling well and could not seem to overcome the nervousness and anxiety that she had been experiencing for quite some time. Three physicians had attributed these symptoms to the death of her husband and to her natural temperament. Her husband had died three years previously. The pesky cough that bothered her "was nothing," she replied to my question about it. Physicians had given her cough medicine and she had gotten some relief, although the cough still persisted. She didn't sleep comfortably at night, either, but then she had always used at least two or three pillows. She had come to me because her daughter, a nurse, had suggested it. "But I am feeling all right," she said. "Things will get better." I asked her if I could listen to her chest and she said, "Sure." When I positioned her on the examining table, I noted several aspects of the way in which she had difficulty getting comfortable and the way her breathing was affected by the slightest exertion. When I listened to her heart and lungs, it was apparent that there was inefficient heart action and that there was fluid in the lung field. I took an electrocardiogram and it verified that there was pathology. I explained this to my client and she asked me to describe to her daughter what I had found. Together, we considered a course of action, and my client decided to see another physician, insisting strongly that it not be one of the doctors she had already seen, because he might get upset. I accompanied her to a different physician, who ordered X rays. The X rays disclosed pleurisy with effusion, and her physician asked her to go to the hospital immediately to have the fluid removed and to undergo tests to ascertain the cause of the lung condition. The final diagnosis was cancer of the lung and liver.

This client had arrived at my office generally representing the categories "*I think* I'm all right . . . but *I wonder*" (what is causing these problems). Again, the physical examination tool and subsequent nursing care led to verification, clarification and decision-making on the part of the client.

Another client example is that of a thirteen-year-old girl whose parents wanted her to have a physical examination performed by me because they were my clients and had come on the recommendation of another client. The young girl was healthy, and she asked only about her flat feet, which sometimes interfered with sports, a favorite activity. On examination of her chest, I heard a murmur through the entire heart cycle over every part of the outline of the heart. The electrocardiogram showed slight aberrations in some of the leads, and on the basis of the murmur I suggested to her and to her parents (with her permission) that she see a cardiologist. His diagnosis was pancake syndrome, which results from a narrow chest cavity and usually disappears at puberty. The case is an example of a client who represents needs in terms of "I'm healthy, with some minor concerns." Nursing care focused on her health assets, emphasizing them as a foundation on which to build and helping to identify some deficits and a course of action for dealing with them.

A fourth client is an example of the category "I know I'm healthy—what can I do to stay that way?" He is a man in his forties whose wife had urged him to see me because he was in the dangerous decade for men with regard to incidence of heart attacks. At the time of his initial appointment the client was and acted the picture of health. He referred to his slight paunchiness, which he lamented from an aesthetic point of view, and he accounted for the foods that caused the excess pounds. "I know what's causing it," he said. "Too much beer and pizza. I used to stop after one or two helpings, but lately I haven't. I don't exercise the way I used to, either. My wife is worried about me, because of the coronary risk factors (which he then proceeded to list). So I told her I would come to have an examination." I did a complete physical examination, including blood work and an EKG. On auscultation of the heart, I identified an increase in his heart rate which I told him occurred when I had the stethoscope over the tricuspid valvular area. He expressed surprise and observed that he was thinking about a problem at work at that point. "Is it possible to have such an immediate alteration in the heart rate? Because that's exactly when I was thinking about work, when you had the stethoscope placed right there. Isn't that amazing?" Nursing care with this client verified his health state and helped him to gain insight into an aspect of himself of which he had been unaware—that pressures of his job could cause an alteration of the heart rate, perhaps indicative that his employment situation should be further explored in an attempt to prevent any health deficits related to the job from developing.

The following example is one in which the client was sure there was illness. The client had been seeing me for nursing assistance aimed at the maintenance of health in the presence of marital difficulty. Her husband subsequently became my client. One evening she called to make an appointment because of some physical symptoms she was experiencing. She was going to see a physician, but her husband suggested that she make an appointment to see me first. When she came to the office she described the following signs and symptoms: In January had a sore throat, which went away and then recurred. No culture was taken. She received penicillin. In the middle of February she felt fatigue and some joint pain. The first of March she felt chills, with no increase in temperature. She was losing weight:

95 pounds, Fall, 1975

93 pounds, December, 1975 (had a physical at the hospital)

95 pounds, January, 1976

92 pounds, March, 1976.

She had lost 1½ inches around her waist and around her hips. Her appetite has been good. Petechiae on R shoulder 3/1/76 lasted until 3/3/76. All joints involved with pain except small joints. Pain is dull, aching, sometimes sharp and throbbing. Worse when pressure is put on joint. No swelling. Prior to 11 A.M. feels fine, after 11 A.M. begins to feel bad. Rests and then starts again for the rest of the day. Sleeps with heating pad, which helps. Hot shower or bath gives relief for a short while. Little relief from aspirin; Phenaphen #3 tried once; relief for a couple of hours. Stomach is "touchy." Is on birth control pills. On Friday, 3/5/76, joints in both hands started to develop pain, off and on, same as other joint pain.

After discussion, she agreed to the steps that I proposed, which were: complete blood count, electrocardiogram, sedimentation rate and a partial examination. On auscultation, I heard a murmur in the apical region of her heart. I suggested that she listen to it, which she did. She decided to see a physician, armed with the results of the laboratory tests, the EKG and the partial physical examination, as well as a list of the symptoms that were important to her. It seems worthy of mention for future discussion that the physician repeated the tests and did a chest X ray although the client pointed out that an X ray had been done a month prior to the appointment with the physician. The significance of this fact will be referred to in a subsequent chapter.

I have used the tool of the physical examination in the way that I use a book as a tool. It has served the purpose of giving me information that I can use in helping my client to make a logical decision about the course of action he or she should pursue. If I were to construct a formula for nursing action in light of my use of the physical examination to achieve nursing goals, it would be this:

> Client's statements + physical examination findings $\longrightarrow$ objective verification of his perspectives of his health state.

No longer am I apprehensive about missing something when I do a partial or complete physical examination of one of my clients. The period of 1971–1976 represents the evolution of the implementation of an idea I had when I started the practice. When I clarified the distinction between the medical goal and the nursing goal in doing a physical examination, I had a feeling much like that of a balloonist when he views the releasing of the last rope holding a balloon to the ground and the balloon floats free!

Perhaps a comment should be made about the nature of my clients' reasons for asking about physical states. Because the content of the chapter pertains to the physical examination, per se, I have confined my discussion to that aspect of the client's needs. It is difficult to discuss the physical examination in isolation, because it is not an isolated technique in my nursing care.

chapter six

Other impressions
as a result of practice

The opening of an independent nursing practice has proved to be the opening of a new world to a nurse who felt professionally corralled in the old one. Each new experience in the past five years has given rise to a multitude of new ideas and impressions. Because they deserve mention, but are not as yet developed enough to warrant separate chapters, I have presented some of them here as "Other Impressions as a Result of Practice." It is hoped that they will prove to be starting points that will lead to further intellectual refinement in the development of professional nursing.

Expressions of need

With the mold broken in terms of the traditional system of caring for one's health state, it was inevitable that new expressions of needs on the part of persons be forthcoming. As I examine the nursing histories of my clients in a very superficial manner, taking only the thread of the needs as presented by my clients, the unusual nature of the reasons why people seek out a nurse can be seen. Before I discuss the types of situations, I would like to warn the reader that I made it clear to the persons seeking my services that I would be approaching their needs from the perspective of nursing care given within a self-care concept. (See Chapter 4.) I emphasized that I am a nurse, not a marriage counselor, social worker, or psychologist, and that I would understand perfectly if they chose to consult another professional in one of those areas. I also assured them that I would constantly be appraising my own expertise and that when I felt that I had reached my limitations, I would tell them that I felt I could no longer be of help. The knowledge that most lay people have has always impressed me. People would respond in such terms as these: (1) I know I could have sought the services of a marriage counselor; as a matter of fact I have seen several in the past, but after a period of time with them I was no longer being helped. I like your approach to me and my problems. (2) Your services are the kind I need, because I know what my problems are—all the others have told me what I already knew about the problem, and I needed to be helped in the way you are helping me. (3) I was trying to tell someone about what you are and what you do, and I couldn't explain it fully. When I said "nurse" they could not understand what I meant, because the image evoked by the word "nurse" is usually seen only in the context of hospitals, clinics, doctors' offices, etc.

Through my practice, I have become aware of the gap that exists in the health care system in the United States, namely that all stages of illness are covered but not all stages of the well state are covered. I believe this gap has emerged because the medical system has been so inflexible in its structure that only when problems reached the point of serious illness and death were any steps taken to investigate the problems. Social, economic, moral and cultural changes should have wrought changes in the ways in which health services could be offered to people living in this climate of change. The big mistake was that even though the professionals in the various fields practiced in light of the changes, the categories of health professionals did not change, and people would line themselves up with the generally understood focus of a particular branch of the health system. As some of my clients have said to me, "Miss Kinlein, I knew I was not mentally ill and yet I needed help. But I didn't need psychological testing. I couldn't get to a clinical psychologist—there are so few—and besides he would have had to work with my physician, and then the inference would have been that I was sick, and I knew I wasn't." One of my clients said she asked her husband, who had been my client prior to marriage, why he hadn't brought her to me earlier, before the situation evolved into such a complicated picture. She felt her decisions would have been far different had she been helped in the way she was being helped by me at the time.

After five years, I have an appreciation of the wide variety of needs that people have in regard to their health states. Although the classification of health professionals is necessary as a step in licensing professional persons, I think it is more important to examine the needs of people and to use those as the point of departure in changing the laws that govern the practice of the particular profession. The people have suffered because of intramural fighting and territorial protection of services. Surely the day has arrived when the needs of the people whom we serve—the real concern of any professional endeavor —should be the measure for determining which service should be provided. The right of the people to choose which persons they will go to for help should be recognized.

The variety of needs expressed to me by clients during the five years of my practice has included: help with a worry, a fear, a concern about the state of health they are in or might be in; help with a marital problem; help with a child; help with pregnancy; help in making a decision about medical care; help in following through on a decision about medical care. These are general categories, and within each there are specific needs as unique as the people expressing them. I can relate the general reasons that have brought people to me for professional nursing, but to explain the particular needs within each generality would be an impossible task at this point. It must always be remembered that it is in transcending the labels—seeing through them, around them and beyond them so that the individual is viewed without presumptions and prejudgments on the part of the nurse—that the essence of professional nursing consists.

Time

As a result of my practice, I have identified *time* as an essential element in giving nursing care. I believe that all nurses have known this for years, but have not been in a position to require that this criterion be met in the traditional settings. I submit that until and unless a provision for the time factor is built into the plans of a nursing department in any setting, good nursing care cannot be given. This means, of course, that demands on the nurse's time arising outside the needs of her client will have to be met by the department under which the needs fall. Good nursing care cannot be fragmented, interrupted and disjointed by the myriad of "activities" traditionally grouped under the title "nursing," and by the helter-skelter routine those tasks impose upon the nurse.

Indeed, I have established that a minimum of one hour—and more often two hours—is needed for the initial appointment between nurse and client. To take a health history (nursing history) in the concept of self-care practices, an hour is required in any setting. The significance of this requirement cannot be overestimated. When a legitimate relationship between nurse and client has been established, the professional nurse should not permit an abridgement of her plan for meeting the needs of the individual who is her client while she is giving nursing care. She should brook no interruption from anyone, and must request that a person interrupting the nurse/client exchange withdraw from their presence. I anticipate a vociferous outcry protesting that this is not possible. In the next chapter, however, I will outline a plan to make it so.

Forms

Because nursing care has not long been given in the setting of the individual practice, it is obvious that it would be premature to develop forms to be used in any aspect of working with the needs or nursing treatment of my clients. One of the universal difficulties with forms in health settings is that the need of the person is structured from without—by the form itself—as opposed to being structured from within the individual. I believe that after I have had 1,000 clients, I will be able to construct guidelines and rules of thumb for other professional nurses to follow. It is likely, however, that nursing may be the only profession that will not be able to collate and use a minimum of information stored on forms in the manner in which other professions can use them. As I have commented, good nursing care cannot depend on and be limited to a careful reading of forms; it must rely on a careful reading of the clients' needs as they are expressed by the clients themselves directly to the professional nurse. Any other approach would negate good nursing care.

In some of my encounters with other professional nurses I have been asked if I have forms that they could use in their work. My response to them has been that it is premature—not to mention hazardous—to use forms as an aid in giving professional nursing care without first having a knowledge of the concept of nursing which will ensure that tools such as forms are placed in the proper perspective. We have too long in nursing put the cart before the horse, allowing techniques to lead our endeavors, leaving the more important conceptual foundations behind in the dust.

The "niceness" of people

The dealings I have had with people in the years of my practice confirm a lifelong belief of mine, namely, that given a chance to be pleasant, understanding, responsive, responsible and honest, 95 percent of the people will display these characteristics. People are aching for a chance to be seen as more virtuous than vicious. And more people scorn dishonesty, deceit and trickery than practice them.

In my practice, I have never been called out at night without good reason. One client called me at eleven in the evening. I talked with her and urged her to call back if necessary, adding, "You know, Mrs. B., I will come to your house to see you." "I know," she responded, "but let me see how I do myself without troubling you to come out here." I urged her to call me as frequently as necessary. She called once more at 1:30 A.M. and then no more. I called her at 7:00 A.M., and she was getting ready to call me to tell me she had improved.

Whenever I have been forced to reschedule an appointment, the clients have always been most understanding. When I ask them what time would be convenient for an appointment, they invariably say, "Whatever time would be convenient for you." They apologize for asking for appointments on weekends and in the evenings. During my practice I have had only one check from a client bounce. That client was also the only one whose behavior made me question whether he had ulterior motives for seeking my services.

My clients have expressed great appreciation for my care and have congratulated me on my endeavor of private practice. The hundreds of clients I have seen have reinforced the positive feelings I have always had for people in general. I believe that a sincere respect for people is a necessary prerequisite to good nursing, for effective professional nursing can ensue only from the conviction that every human being is unique and important, that what he says and what he feels is worthy of attention and should be taken seriously by the professional nurse. On this basis mutual respect grows, and the resulting rapport between nurse and client works to the benefit of both.

Nature of relationships

In my practice, one of the most important differentiations that had to be made concerned the nature of the relationships established with the persons who came to me for professional care. The fine line that most other professionals in other fields had been coping with for many decades I now experienced for the first time in my nursing career. Friends came to me for nursing, and strangers came to me for nursing; some of these strangers have become very close friends.

In the early days, when my security lay primarily in the areas of traditional nursing episodes and situations, I felt very humble when friends who are nurses came to me with trust—their knowledge and mine came essentially from curricula formed in the mold required by one universal standard, State Board examinations. There was a degree of apprehension and a feeling of "no underfooting" when I was confronted with needs that did not require "doing for." In hospitals I had cared for nurses without a second thought; now, the setting was changed, and I was giving nursing care in a new and different framework. *The nurses approached me in an exceptionally confidence-inspiring manner, and I shall always be grateful to each and every professional nurse who is or who has been my client.* However, in my capacity as a professional nurse I moved quickly into giving nursing care and forgot all else, except to try my utmost to help the person who was my client. I identified this feeling with my very first client, who is a professional nurse; it was not until she had left that I fully realized that I had my first client and that she was a professional nurse. (See the Appendix for her nursing needs.)

A second type of relationship involves the stranger who is not a nurse and whose care presents such a challenge that wholly unorthodox methods of giving care must be devised. The innovative methods of giving therapeutic nursing care call for an extremely fine line to be established in judging the effect the nursing action will have on the client. An example will serve to make the point.

One of my clients, to be cited again in the following chapter, is a 46-year-old retarded man. Because the approach to him through the years has been a medical one, the emphasis has been on his limitations, on what he cannot do, on the degree of his retardation. His sister initially requested my services for him and thought it best to tell him that a friend was coming to visit. I made my first contact with him on a house call to his apartment, where he lives alone. Immediately, I introduced myself as a professional nurse. I had to establish a relationship that would not be proceeding from the pathological aspect of his condition, even though he asked questions about the nature of my nursing care from the medical perspective. "I'm not sick now," he would say with a laugh, in a mildly protesting way. I would explain that as a professional nurse I looked at how well people are when I care for them. "Not many nurses do that kind of nursing," was his astute observation. Initially, he was not very discriminating about the number of times he called me at the office and at the apartment. Now, he distinguishes between his contacts with me that are professional ones helping him in the exercise of his self-care agency and contacts that are classified as nonprofessional. My professional contacts with him include discussion of matters about his family relationships, his eating practices and other self-care measures. The professional contacts also include structuring a social setting in which bantering and teasing go on. On these occasions, I invite understanding friends to lunch or dinner in a restaurant with us, and thus the circle of people with whom he can exchange words and ideas is enlarged. At all times, control is maintained by me in a professional manner, even if the tone is light and social. Through careful use of social situations my client is helped to grow in ways that are different from the social development occurring in his family circle—ways which constitute a special contribution to his growth.

In these matters, I am aware of the fact that one of the most difficult situations for the retarded person to manage is one of controlled social intercourse. Because the number of people who can relate to him on a basis of friendship are few, and because the degree of friendship that accompanies professional nursing care can fill a void in the person's life, frequently any gesture of friendship can be abused and overused by that person. This fact used to be viewed as a burden that interferes with care in the minds of some nurses, instead of being seen as a point of departure for giving nursing care. I believe this nursing need can be met best in the independent practice setting simply because of the necessity of tailoring the care to the need expressed by each individual who bears the medical diagnosis of retardation. The professional nurse must, of course, exercise sound judgment in such cases, but that is, after all, the hallmark of the professional nurse.

Nurses' reactions

The reception accorded to my ideas by groups of professional nurses and nursing students is an indication that the time is ripe for change in the field of nursing. One illustration in particular has left the professional nurses who hear me speak nodding their heads in affirmation. In it I describe the differences between night nursing, evening nursing and day nursing that I experienced in the late 40s, 50s and 60s.

When I was caring for people during the time period from 11 P.M. to 7 A.M. I was continuously under a unique pressure. If the condition of Mrs. X changed, I would study the medical record, check what had occurred in surgery, examine the laboratory reports and conduct a physical examination—auscultation of her heart and lungs, palpation of her abdomen—double-checking constantly, over what I had to decide was a "safe" period of time to wait, before calling the intern on duty. My physical state at this time would show tachycardia, perspiring palms and a sense of stress. If I decided to call the intern, and if my call proved necessary—because medical intervention in Mrs. X's condition was required—I was a "good nurse." If my call turned out to be unnecessary, then I was not a "good nurse."

From 7 A.M. to 3 P.M. I would put away the instruments I had been expected to use at night to make sound judgments, or I would have been subjected to sarcastic comments accusing me of being a "little doctor." And I proceeded to do what nurses on the day shift do—give baths, distribute medications, carry out prescribed treatments (and in so doing I knew I was carrying out the technical aspects of the medical care)—because there were many physicians present during the day period, and thus my judgments were clearly made to seem inappropriate.

From 3 P.M. until 11 P.M., when the physicians left, I would let one intellectual "antenna" at a time become operable as one physician after another disappeared. Finally, at midnight, all of my intellectual "antennae" were vibrating wildly, and I would be in the same stressful state again. *It became clear to me that I was then a doctor substitute.* Yet, I had chosen to be a nurse, not a physician.

Whenever I recount this example, by way of illustrating the clear understanding I now have of knowing what nursing is, the response of professional nurses and junior- and senior-year learners of nursing shows overwhelming agreement —as evidenced by their applause.

What is the significance of this example 30

years after I experienced it? The fact that it is poignant to today's young nurses illustrates that nursing schools and nursing departments in service settings have done little to clarify *what nursing is*. Through all those years, nothing much has changed.

Two questions thrust themselves upon our consciousness:

1. Is the care in hospital settings third-rate medicine, in terms of:

   Physicians, 7 A.M. to 3 P.M.

   Residents and interns, 7 A.M. to 3 P.M.; 3 P.M. to 11 P.M.

   Professional nurses, 11 P.M. to 7 A.M.

2. Is justice being violated when demands are made on the professional nurse that presume a level of knowledge operative at a certain point in time, the application of which knowledge at any other point in time is likely to precipitate wiltingly sarcastic comments that shake her faith in herself and her self-image?

As a professional nurse client of mine commented to me, "It's so hard in the clinical situation. You are continually under the pressure of deciding whether you were aggressive enough, not aggressive enough, or too aggressive in regard to action taken in the absence of the physician. You either get told, 'You're stupid. Why in hell didn't you call me sooner?' Or you are told, 'You are taking over the practice of medicine.'"

This type of situation—including similar comments—was what gave me so much distress when I was in the traditional settings. That time period was in the fifties and sixties, the pressure being worse in the sixties. In addition, when a professional nurse wants to (but may not) take action on the basis of knowledge substantiated in scientific fact and literature; and when she is powerless to act when action is taken contrary to that knowledge base, I denounce a system that compels her to choose between standing by and watching the resultant setback to the patient or taking interceptive action at the risk of reprisal in some form—and of a lingering air of hostility directed at her.

The churning discomfort that prevailed in the traditional settings is a sharp contrast to the serenity I have experienced in the last five years. In my practice of nursing in the independent setting, I have been overwhelmed by the pure joy that comes with nursing. The challenge that I so welcomed, the zestful feeling I experienced with every call from a client— how I yearn to convey it adequately to my professional nursing colleagues!

Often I have been asked how my nursing colleagues accept me in the role of independent practitioner. My response is that initially the lay people moved very quickly in accepting me—as evidenced by comments asking why nurses have waited so long to make themselves available; or expressing frustration that the only way to obtain nursing care in the past has been to be ill, see a doctor and be hospitalized. Others have remarked that they are satisfied with their medical care; they have a good doctor; but to help them now, they need a nurse. In retrospect, it has sometimes been difficult for professional nurses to accept as nursing the care that I give to people in my practice. Time and again they attempt to put a label on it, such as "basically interviewing," "really just listening," "actually a facilitator," "public health nursing," "mental health (or psychiatric) nursing," "counseling." My response has been, "But why does a label other than nursing have to be put on it?"

My interpretation of these responses to my nursing care has been that the average nurse does not have a balanced view of what she can give from a professional perspective, and that this partial view constitutes an implicit denigration of the value and worthiness of nursing.

A group of nurses have supported me from the beginning, nurses who seemed to have an unusual degree of insight into the value of my endeavor. A small group of physicians have expressed congratulations and interest in my endeavor. After five years, it is my impression that there is a revolutionary movement afoot in the nursing world. Now, when nurses hear about what I have done, there is an excitement generated that I assess as a prelude to concerted action. Prior to last year, there were some skepticism and at times rejection on the part of individual nurses who appraised my practice. I predict that a major change is brewing in the nursing field that is unique in terms of other changes that have taken place over the years in nursing. Needless to say, I encourage and will aid and abet any change that calls for the autonomous practice of professional nursing in any setting.

Perception of nurses

If change in the practice of nursing is to come about, of course, it must be accompanied by a change in the perception of nurses by other members of the health professions.

I recall one experience in particular that illustrates the low esteem in which nurses are held by some in the health field. I went to a hospital one day to read the medical record of a client, at the client's request. One person in the records room, who explained she was "not in charge," was extremely pleasant and helpful and obtained the chart for me, after I presented the proper identification and the signed form giving permission to me from my client. Another person, who was in charge, was quite the opposite in her manner. When she entered the room, the first person explained to her that I was a professional nurse asking to read the records of a client who had been a patient in the hospital. The second person did not greet me, frowned at me and said, "What do you want? Who are you?" I introduced myself by name and title and explained again that I was in independent practice and that one of my clients had asked me to look at her medical record; I again showed the signed permission form and compared the signature with the one on the medical record.

"Could I have the chart back?" she responded, holding out her hand. "I'll have to check with the doctor."

I gave her the chart, saying pleasantly, "I don't think it's necessary to check with the doctor. My client has given me her permission."

"Oh, yes, it is," she said in a most disagreeable tone.

I sat in a booth in the records room while she called the doctor's office from a telephone a few feet away from me. The conversation went like this:

"Look, there's a professional nurse here who wants to look at a patient's record. No, not from the hospital here. She said she has her own practice. . . . yeah. . . . in Hyattsville. Says on her paper, here, 'office visits and house calls by appointment.' . . . No, neither have I. . . . yeah, the patient signed the permission form, but I thought Dr. ——— ought to know. (some low, inaudible words) I don't know. She has five doctors. . . . yeah. . . . well, OK, tell the doctor, will you? Thanks."

She leaned back in her chair and said, "If another doctor wanted to look at the chart, I'd have to let the doctor know."

I replied, "Yes, I can understand that would be necessary."

"Besides," she added, "we have to have two days' notice to get it and all. You know, this record belongs to the hospital. The content is the patient's, but it is the property of the hospital."

I spoke strongly, "The content of the record belongs to the individual."

"Yes, that's true," she said testily. "But the chart is the hospital's. You can come back on Friday between 9:30 and 10:00, and if it's all right, you can look at it then."

I essayed a comment that I thought would be helpful: "I can understand why this is a difficult idea for you, because it is a new idea for nursing. . . . You see, . . ."

"Oh, I understand about nursing," she interrupted.

There are many perceptual barriers that must be overcome whenever new concepts and practices are developed. In nursing, the barriers are fortified by tradition and stereotype. There is a twofold responsibility involved here: It remains a large and arduous task for those seeking to initiate change to help others to understand by exercising patience, courtesy and professionalism—but also strength. It is the duty of those professionals steeped in the established order of things to keep a mental door open to the entrance of new ideas and to meet them with respect and creative, critical (not cynical) inquisitiveness. Those of us whose livelihoods are involved with the health and welfare of other human beings must remember to judge new concepts and suggested changes in terms of how they benefit those people—our real masters—and not in terms of how they threaten the established routine—the false master that all too often rules the health professions.

Approach to individuals

A comment must be made about the approach to individuals and their health state used by nurses in the traditional settings. I am reminded of an instance in which a two-year-old client of mine had to have immunization injections. Her grandparents had brought her to me for nursing care and for an assessment of her health state. It was time for immunizations, so I made the appropriate arrangements at the county clinic for her to receive the injections. On the telephone, I had indicated that she was in good health.

When the grandparents and I arrived at the clinic, the nurse got out the form for the history and I answered all the questions in the negative. I said, "She has not had any illnesses at all." The nurse said, "She hasn't had any illness, has not been sick at all?" "No," I responded. The nurse then went down the list of diseases, asking if the child had had any, and I kept replying "No, no, no. . . ." The nurse then turned to the grandmother and asked her if the child had ever been ill, and the grandmother answered no. Again, the nurse went down the list of diseases and the grandmother responded exactly as I had responded. The grandmother commented to me "how unnecessary" the repetition had been.

With the current nursing orientation toward abnormal conditions, and with the unfortunate emphasis that only a doctor's word can be accepted (and not, incidentally, a professional nurse's) in regard to the state of health of people, the net result for the client is that he is regarded as not really knowing anything. The obvious question arises, What about the person who will deliberately lie for some reason about his state of health? And the next question must be, How can repeated questioning of him—by a nurse, a doctor or anyone—disclose the prevarication after all is said and done? This approach also makes the person appear to be incapable of taking care of himself in so simple a matter as being able to report what illnesses he has suffered. If the need is felt by the nurse to pursue questioning to the point of repetitiveness so that she will not subsequently be blamed for failing to relay medical information to the doctor—so that *he* will be prevented from making an error in the administration of medication to the patient—then I submit that the nurse is functioning clearly as an extension of the physician. The net result is that, in the eyes of the person being questioned, the nurse's behavior is lacking in logic and/or that the physician is a benevolent tyrant, expecting (and for the most part getting) service by professionals that accrues to his prestige and supports his claims of practicing expertly and without error.

Medical science

The needs my clients have expressed leave open to a great deal of debate the state of medical science in handling a multiplicity of "minor," "vague" complaints on the part of the client. In the words of my clients, "You have to be really sick before the medical profession can help you these days." Yet "minor," "vague" complaints can arouse anxiety in the client when they are not understood; and thus needs emerge that for years have gone unmet. Such complaints can tell the client much about his total health state before they manifest themselves in pathological signs that can be objectively spotted by a professional. For years we may have been missing the first and vital clues to impending illness simply because we have not been listening hard enough to perceive them.

What confronts the thinking person at this point is the question of comparison of medical care rendered in the past and in the present. Is it possible that the sympathy, companionship, care and concern of the old-time family practitioner was in reality a mobilizing pivot for the family? Can, indeed, the question legitimately be asked, Did the nature of medical cures in the early part of the century lie in the fact of self-action on the part of the patient and his family? If not, then *where are the cures in a medical science frame of reference for the common diseases, the "minor illnesses," the "that's to be expected" category of illness?* Is it possible that medicine's justified orientation to dramatic cures for more unusual or life threatening diseases has left unattended a whole host of more common, annoying and partly incapacitating conditions? Is it possible that another discipline could shed light on the nature of physiological alterations? Would this contribute to a reversal of the health picture of many Americans? Should we look at the fact that "nature" accomplishes 90 percent of the cure? Is it possible that the approach to investigation and research into the diseases and illness that plague us has been at the wrong end of the spectrum? If 1,000,000 professional nurses shifted their focus in caring for people to the perspective of "how well are you?" could we reverse the process of illness? A physician may state: "All this health orientation in the nursing field is fine, but we need help in taking care of a lot of sick people. Therefore, the curriculum in schools of nursing should be emphasizing the technical care of sick people." And we must ask ourselves, Does this make sense?

Education

The fact that in my practice I have gleaned data directly from the clients without a preexisting bias about their needs carries tremendous implications regarding the methods of and approach to the teaching of nursing in universities. The uniqueness of the situation—in which the professional nurse is really controlling the direction of the care in meeting the needs expressed by the clients—shifts the emphasis away from teaching what has been done in the past in nursing to developing the ability of the nurse to make sound judgments in light of what she is confronted with as each client communicates with her.

This basic difference between what nursing has been and what nursing can be should provide nursing educators with a significant challenge—and a topic for serious consideration, study and debate—as they strive to design programs that truly prepare nurses for the *professional* roles they should be filling in the health system.

chapter seven

Steps to effect change in the health system

Before change can occur in the way nursing care is given in both traditional and new settings, a change must be effected in the total approach to health care in the United States. Presently the system of nursing care is seen as part of the overall medical care of a person. Were this not true I would not have the hundreds of examples which verify that I was indeed breaking tradition by being alone in my nursing practice.

One of these experiences occurred as recently as April, 1976, when one of my clients made an appointment with a specialist. She later described the encounter to me. The specialist asked her the name of her family doctor. She replied that she had none. "But you have to have a doctor," the specialist said. "I need to talk to him about your condition." Again, the client said that she had no doctor. "Well, I have to tell a doctor about your heart condition," the specialist continued. "It has to be recorded in your medical file." My client responded, "The person who knows the most about my general condition and who has given me good nursing care is Miss Kinlein, who has her own office. I've been going to her for four years now." The physician's response was classic—and revealed a great deal about nursing in the current health care system. "Oh, she has to have a doctor with her. She can't be alone. She has to be with a doctor." After relating the experience to me, my client said, "Miss Kinlein, it is futile to tell these guys about a nurse who gives nursing care and helps the patient to make decisions about her general health state. And it's useless to ask them to comply with my request to have them send you my medical records. I want you to have them. They won't send them."

It is obvious that a distinction must be made between a medical system that controls all aspects of a person's health state and a true health system, which permits freedom of movement on the part of the person seeking professional help in the system. I would like to propose a system in which medical care is but a part of the total health system, along with other systems, such as nursing, nutrition, health education, psychology, etc.

In speaking of a health system, one must avoid the pitfall of equating it with a medical system; the terms must not be considered interchangeable. The notion that a health system embraces many subsystems, one of which is a medical care system, is a more accurate concept. This concept is a more logical one, since the definition of health as prevention of disease is unacceptable; whereas the positive approach of maintaining a healthy state and improving on the total health of a person *is* acceptable. Therefore, the point of departure in planning to meet health needs must not be an ill state, or even the prevention of an ill state. If no disease can be identified, is the person therefore "healthy" and excluded from the health care system? This is the question that must be looked at, if the medical approach is used in planning for health. Since, philosophically speaking, the formal object of medicine is disease—the diagnosis and treatment thereof—then a medical system cannot be viewed as a health system; for the mode of entry into the system involves an appraisal that presupposes the presence of illness or disease—or, in some cases, screening for early signs and symptoms premonitory of a disease state.

I would like to propose a health care system in which the person is the primary giver of care to himself—by virtue of choosing the health professional who he thinks would be most helpful to him at the time—and in which the health professional would proceed to assist the individual, in his own field of expertise—making recommendations for other expert opinions and care when appropriate. The chameleon-like nature and degree of the needs of people stand out in sharp contrast to the unrelieved rigidity of disease classification and pathologic processes. Since we health professionals are not intellectual chameleons, one set of health workers cannot presume to have the knowledge and skill to identify, let alone meet, all the varying needs of the individual in meeting his health goals. The era of public ignorance about physiology, psychology and disease is past. People now want verification and expansion of their knowledge base and of their self-care practices, and they want assistance in making decisions that affect their health states. These needs are a step beyond the public education that results from material presented in the various mass media, and they demand individual attention as the person becomes a self-care agent in light of his unique attributes and health characteristics. Such are the needs of my clients as they decide to seek my services as a professional nurse. The discrete disciplines of anatomy and physiology, biochemistry, electrophysiology, pharmacology and pathology are drawn upon by many professionals with different goals in mind; the identification and achievement of these goals by the various professional practitioners become the sine qua non of any professional practice discipline. To suppose that the use of knowledge of pathology is automatically going to evolve into a medical diagnosis is to make an erroneous assumption.

Again, it must be remembered that a concept of nursing can relate to self-care practices in regard to a state of health—plus the science of human physiology, plus the client who has a need for nursing in regard to his self-care practices. The process thus represents a unified concept, in which physiology is *the* scientific discipline, fused with the concept of self-care practices in regard to a state of health, in the practice discipline of nursing.

So, I am proposing a system of health care in which the client is the person who selects the professional practitioner for his primary care. His needs determine the structure of the health system, which will now make *all* the health professionals available to him, *initially, in all settings*, both traditional settings and new ones yet to be designed. For the nursing professional, it would be the equivalent of turning a glove completely inside out to offer to the public for the first time all the ability, talent and concern that nurses have always had, but which was unseen because the contribution of the nurse to the person was filtered through the system. At last, all the expertise of nursing could be presented as an entity to the individual needing nursing care. At last, the client would see the nurse as an extension of himself and not as an extension of the physician.

If such a health system were put into effect in the United States, then the next logical step would be to make available to all health professionals the use of facilities that would enable them to accomplish the goals peculiar to the specific professions. From my practice, I can identify instances in which I believe the person's health could be maintained and improved if there existed facilities to which he or she could be admitted for nursing care. Implicit in such an arrangement would be the need to have clearly identified goals, so that a time interval and personnel needs could be projected. Here are three examples:

1. The parents of a four-year-old boy with a diagnosis of Down's syndrome needed help in regard to the child's dietary practices. He needed 24-hour nursing care in order to establish nutritionally sound dietary practices. If he could be admitted to a hospital for nursing care aimed at establishing such patterns, the parents—and the child—would be helped immeasurably in maintaining and improving the total health state of the child and, since the child's progress affects others, the total health state of the family.

2. I have a 78-year-old client who lives alone and is in reasonably good health. About three times a year, I would like to admit her to an institution for rest and assistance in self-care practices, such as nutrition. She does well through the year; and such nursing admissions would provide her with concentrated nursing care to help her stay healthy and get even healthier.

3. Another client is a 46-year-old man who is mildly retarded. He has a job at the post office and lives in an apartment by himself. His family is devoted to him and is very helpful to

him. With the professional nursing care that he has been receiving he is disclosing hidden abilities for understanding and participating in conversations with ease, and he demonstrates to a marked degree a wit that flows from an ability to discern nuances of meaning. There has been steady progress in his development and performance of self-care measures, and if he could be admitted to an institution for specified periods several times a year, for a precisely designed course of nursing measures, I believe he could accomplish even more.

The basic principle involved in these situations is that there should exist facilities devoted to meeting the *health* needs of individuals, as well as the *medical* needs; to helping people *remain* well, in addition to helping people *get* well.

Even in the traditional hospital setting, however, where the focus is usually to cure or control disease, there is room for the professional nurse practicing independently. A person who is admitted to a hospital has anxieties, concerns and needs that remain unrelieved by the cadre of nurses, aides and technicians who approach him with an isolated and specific concern, such as taking blood pressure, removing a bed pan, taking blood, etc. However, there is no one professional accountable to the patient who considers the totality of the person occupying bed number such-and-such in room number such-and-such. In the hospital setting, the person may not understand what is being done to him, or why; he may need help in making decisions that must be made quickly, may need help accepting or adjusting to a diagnosis and prognosis. But that is only the beginning. We have no way of knowing now which of the many kinds of needs peculiar to individuals are involved when a given person enters the hospital setting, because heretofore the needs have been unexplored, unrecognized and, of course, unfulfilled. However, a professional nurse acting as the extension of the person in a hospital setting could do much to maintain health by working with such needs, while the medical needs were being taken care of by those responsible for them.

If such nursing care is to be available in hospitals, of course, there must be a drastic revision of the present organizational structure and policies of those institutions. In any revision, provision must be made for the features of availability, accessibility, accuracy, accountability and autonomy* to be implemented. When I have been asked if it is possible to have these features observed in the hospital setting, I have responded in the affirmative. The next inevitable question is, "How is it possible?" When I gave a workshop to the nursing staff at the Georgetown University Medical Center Hospital in 1975, I disclosed for the first time a plan to make it possible. To the credit of Meriam Van Eron, the basic plan has been initiated on one unit, and the results will undoubtedly appear in the literature at some future date.

The following is a blueprint for action allowing professional nursing care to be given in the hospital setting:

A person coming to the hospital can, if he desires, have access to a professional nurse who practices within a concept of nursing and who can effect a legitimate nurse-client relationship. This contact will be the first one made upon entering the hospital, literally at the door to the hospital, before the person goes to the admitting office or anywhere else. At this time, the professional nurse will meet with the person to determine with him if he wants and needs nursing care and to assess the nature of his nursing needs. A list of professional nurses who are willing and able to establish legitimate nursing relationships would be available to the person seeking such nursing care. From that point on during his hospitalization the person would have that professional nurse accountable to him (the fee for services to be paid by the person as an item separate from the overall charges of the hospital); *the hospital charges would reflect the subtraction of the cost for nursing care that is presently built into the charges for hospitalization regardless of the needs of the patients and their desires in regard to nursing care.* The professional nurse with whom the person has established a legitimate nurse-client relationship would design a nursing system for that person and would direct and control it while he is hospitalized. *If the person does not desire such nursing care, or if the nurse determines it is not nursing care that is expected and*

---

* The characteristics of professionalism discussed in Chapter 3.

desired, the responsibility for the care of that person comes under the appropriate department—medicine, dietary, etc. At any point during his hospitalization, the person can request nursing care under the direction of a professional nurse. The decisions regarding nursing care must be put in the hands of professional nurses, in or out of the traditional health settings.

The availability of such nursing care is explained to the prospective hospital patient in this way:

When you come to the hospital, a professional nurse will greet you and take you to a room where she will talk with you, in order to ascertain whether you want or need professional nursing care during your hospital stay; you will then make the decision whether or not to choose a professional nurse, who will be your nurse in a legitimate nurse-client relationship. This professional nurse will be *your* nurse in the same manner that the physician is *your* doctor, or a lawyer is *your* lawyer, etc. The professional nurse you choose will assume full responsibility for your nursing care and will design, control and implement the system of nursing care while you are in the hospital and for as long as there is mutual agreement to continue the professional relationship. A fee will be paid to the professional nurse, and the cost of any nonprofessional nursing care (which will be controlled by the professional nurse) will be itemized on your hospital bill and clearly separated from the other costs of hospitalization. If you decide not to have professional nursing care at the beginning of your stay in the hospital, but subsequently decide to engage the services of a professional nurse, you will be able to contact the nurse who greeted you or another professional nurse of your choice. This system of providing nursing care should not be confused with the arrangement of private duty nursing or special duty nursing care given in the traditional manner.

It would seem that if an institution were to conduct an experimental study to ascertain the wishes of the people in regard to receiving nursing care, the results would show that nursing has moved a giant step toward the acquisition of professional stature in the eyes of the public. Obviously, valid inferences could be made, in light of the findings, in regard to cost factors of hospitalization, improved health care while in the hospital (and when the person returns home), identification of the kinds of needs people have when they are hospitalized and guidelines for the future in terms of facilities for providing care in the health system.

Prerequisite to such care, of course, would be the proper education of nurses regarding a concept of nursing care and acceptance of the notion of being able to practice nursing independently in any setting. The idea that I have just proposed has been well received by the majority of professional nurses who have taken my courses or who have heard me speak. They have seen the value of such experimentation and their questions are action-oriented, indicating that they have moved past the stage of accepting the idea.

Such changes also call for additional education of the public regarding the role that professional nursing can play in their total health states—in or out of the hospital setting—and the roles of other health professionals with whom the professional nurse will come into contact on behalf of her clients.

If ever there was a need for change in an existing institution, so that good nursing care could be given, the need exists in the institution known as the nursing home. Changes must be effected not only in the organizational structure and policies of nursing homes, but also in the laws governing their administration. In order that the magnitude of the problem may be appreciated, it is necessary to trace a bit of the history of nursing homes.

Initially, nursing homes for the most part (although there are always exceptions) were operated in a scandalous manner. The persons admitted to the homes were treated as inanimate objects to be kept alive so that money could be obtained for their "care." As society changed, and the sons, daughters and other relatives of the elderly had no means of caring for their aging loved ones, nursing homes mushroomed. It was necessary to control the "care" that was given, and regulation of the homes was a good thing. Unfortunately, the methods of regulating them were determined by physicians, who had only a medical perspective from which to proceed in planning. So they planned for the medical care in nursing homes. Also unfortunately, nurses did not have an articulated concept of nursing, so that caring for people in nursing homes became easy, in the sense that much of the pressure of acute care as well as the responsibility given to nurses in the acute settings was absent. There was a degree of peace and serenity in the atmosphere of the nursing home, and the pace was much less hectic. There was an absence of challenge to the physician and a lack of judgments to be rendered, since there were no complex diagnoses to be made and no attending complex therapies to be prescribed. The value of the care given in this setting was seen to be very low. "After all," the reasoning went, "there is nothing to do in a nursing home except to keep the patients clean and give out pills." Such distorted thinking about the complexities involved in every situation in which human beings are caring for human beings produced the dismal result guaranteed by such an approach. It supported the notion that nursing was not worth much—that the only care of value in the health field was medical care. Also, in a system in which the professional nurse acted as a substitute for the absent physician in giving out the many medications, and in which the pay scale was less than the minimum wage in many instances, the persons nursing the aging loved ones of families were at best young and inexperienced—but eager to help and to serve—and at worst lazy, disgruntled, discourteous and heady with the power that comes when a helpless individual is completely in another's hands.

As of today, progress has been made toward the improvement of the situation described above. But now, nursing homes that try to improve the nursing care they give are finding their hands tied by legislation that does not permit nurses to give nursing care, but allows them to act only as keepers of the system for state and federal governments. The problem that is currently before the public concerning the lack of good care of nursing home residents seems to have an obvious solution—so obvious that one wonders if the whole point has been missed and somewhere beneath all the logic and obviousness of the situation there lurks a Hydra, successfully defeating all attempts to eliminate its menace.

Lest anyone conclude erroneously that I speak from less than firsthand experience, I note that I have "worked" in a nursing home and that in light of the concept of nursing I had developed at that point, I took action to preserve the responsibility that I had as a professional nurse in making decisions about the nursing care of an individual. One of the times I took action was in the case of a sixty-five-year-old woman with arthrosed joints from arthritis and with many decubiti. She was perfectly rational; indeed she had a sense of humor which she readily displayed. She always said how much better she felt after she had been turned (at two-hour intervals throughout the night) and had taken a drink of water. She would thank the nursing aide and me, and soon she would fall asleep, only to wake up in pain and discomfort and ask to be turned again. One night I noticed that the physician had written on her chart, "Do not turn this patient." I thought he had made a mistake and had put the notation on the wrong chart, and I continued to turn her. One month later the same notation was on the woman's chart, this time taking up several lines, for emphasis. I found it hard to believe that a physician would write this medical prescription in 1970, when so much had been researched about bed rest and the deterioration of the body because of immobility. I tried to contact the physician during the day (I worked nights), but was unsuccessful. I continued to turn the woman. (I had informed the director of nursing that I intended to turn her and to continue with my nursing care.) One month later, the same notation appeared, taking up the whole sheet. I investigated and learned that the practical nurse who specialed this person on days had complained to the doctor that I was not giving enough Demerol at night, that her patient was uncomfortable because she had been turned so much during the night, and that it was very difficult to make her comfortable during the day. I had had it. I sat down and wrote on the chart for anyone and everyone to see: "Because the physician is interfering with my nursing care, I will no longer take responsibility for this resident." I then added a full explanation. I did not take care of that resident any longer at night; the aides gave her what care she needed.

Legislation should aim at the support of the large group of professional nurses who have as their chief concern the welfare of persons who need care. In other words, the law should make it possible for nurses to set standards, arrange for methods of evaluation and insure the observance of good nursing care in the homes. After all, there is significance in the word *nursing* in the institution known as a nursing home. Those most deserving of better pay—those who actually give the care to the persons in nursing homes—should receive it. In regard to the nature of the giving of care in nursing homes, it must be admitted that tediousness is its most outstanding aspect. Because such care demands patience, creativity and an ability to guard against letting it become "routine," the need for a professional approach is more pressing.

My blueprint for change in the nursing home setting calls for a situation in which the resident and relatives would select a professional nurse in the same way that they choose a particular lawyer, physician, etc. The professional nurse, who must have a concept of nursing care, accepts the family as her clients. The fees are paid directly to the nurse for nursing care; the family contracts with the institution for supportive services. Nursing has to be free of restrictions in order to render the best of its services to the public. In addition, with the emphasis on what is strong and right with the resident—as opposed to approaching him from the perspective of illness, or of what is wrong with him—it is possible that the statistics concerning the use of some, but not all, of their capacities by our aged population and by the general population would be drastically revised.

One of the best examples of good nursing care and its effectiveness is Collingswood Nursing Center in Rockville, Maryland, with its able nurse administrator, Mrs. Roxanne Stigers. One of my clients, Mr. N., presents a case in point.

Mr. N. is a 66-year-old man with a medical diagnosis of Alzheimer's disease. He was admitted to a nursing home for two and a half months. Because the nursing staff had a medical orientation, as opposed to a nursing orientation, in the care of the people in the home, my client was given large daily doses of Thorazine, and the monthly bill for this and other medications was very heavy. Furthermore, Mr. N.'s condition involved complete loss of control of urine, feces, and saliva, and he sat in his chair all day until bedtime.

Mrs. N. was advised that because of her husband's aggressiveness and hitting out at people in the home, it was imperative that he be admitted to a state mental institution. The medical forms had been signed by a psychiatrist and were awaiting the signature of another physician when Mrs. N. took him out of the nursing home and kept him at home until a bed was available at Collingswood. Mrs. Stigers and I worked together in giving care to Mr. N. from an administrative perspective as well as in regard to the actual nursing care. Now Mr. N. presents this picture: he is on much lighter doses of Valium; he goes out for walks and dinner with his wife and family; he has urinary and bowel control *when explicit nursing measures are followed;* he is not resistive or abusive *when explicit nursing measures are followed.* His wife is delighted because, as she says, "He is so happy; I can tell." It is important to note that because of the relationship between the physician, who is at present the medical director at Collingswood, and Mrs. Stigers and me, we three functioned in the true sense of colleagues, and the care of Mr. N. continues to be effective at Collingswood.

An example of the type of input that a professional nurse can contribute in a situation such as the one described above can be seen in the following nursing system designed by me for Mr. N. and presented to Mrs. Stigers.

Design of Nursing System for Mr. J. N.

In light of Mr. N.'s medical diagnosis of Alzheimer's disease, it would seem that the design of the nursing system for him should be based on the following facts:

1. His attention span is about 10 seconds.

2. His ability to comprehend an idea is at the minimal level.

3. His ability to convey his right to refuse is at the subarticulate level; hence he will manifest his responses through physical gestures and application of his physical strength.

4. Further, his ability to understand any reasoning on the part of another person depends on the use of gentle tones by that person, not on the logic of words.

5. Moreover, he will not *grow* in understanding, because he does not have the capacity to grow and develop mentally.

6. Multiple stimuli simultaneously confronting Mr. N. will confuse, disturb, and frighten him.

7. Loud noises and heightened activity in his immediate surroundings will agitate him.

8. Any *small* change in any part of his care will make him feel insecure.

Therefore, the nursing procedures should be:

1. *Identically* carried out each time, even if the nursing personnel changes.

2. Only one person at a time should be in direct contact with Mr. N.

3. Careful notations should be made concerning changes in his behavior so that accurate modifications of the regimen can be made, to insure the best results.

I would like to prescribe, then, the following steps in the nursing care of Mr. N.:

1. The explicit setting forth of the detailed steps in his care.

For example:

a) Approach Mr. N. with a relaxed manner, smile, and then greet him.

b) Speak slowly, in a subdued tone of voice.

c) Say: "Here is your wash cloth . . . (pause). Wash your face, Mr. N." (Wait ten seconds. Repeat the same words in the same tone.)

d) Turn your attention to something else. Do not talk to Mr. N.

e) Then go back to him and if necessary, repeat the above.

Mrs. ——— will write up the steps she uses in caring for Mr. N. during the daytime. It is suggested that one person write up the detailed steps of his/her approach to Mr. N. for the evenings and nights. Each person should follow these steps exactly, in the absence of the persons who wrote the steps.

Mrs. N.'s participation in the care of her husband should also be incorporated, so the nursing chart should look like this:

Steps to be Followed	*Mrs. N.'s Comments*

(My nursing measures were supplemented with information from Mrs. N. about the habits and behavior of her husband.)

No further detail about Mr. N.'s case is needed, to show how the professional nurse, working with other health professionals and the client's family, acted to insure the good care of her client in the nursing center.

In general, nursing homes should be re-analyzed in light of the following points:

The care in a nursing home demands that the giver of nursing care be self-disciplined, mature and knowledgeable. Justice demands that monetary recognition be given to those who meet these demands and who give good care on a continuing basis, so that the dreadful picture of nursing homes in the United States can be remedied. These questions must be addressed: *Is the criterion of absence of complexity in medical care a valid basis for perpetuating the system that now exists? Since nurses now notify the physician when medical care is needed, should not the system be changed so that it is organizationally obvious that medical care is secondary to the nursing care that the residents receive in nursing homes? Since it can be demonstrated that nursing care in nursing homes is complex, should not the system support the nurse from the moral, legal and financial perspectives?*

The suggested changes in this chapter deserve discussion and consideration by all those who determine and implement policy in the existing health institutions in the country. Such institutions—dedicated to the health and welfare of human beings—should not rest complacently on tradition when the opportunity exists for even better care of the persons whose lives are entrusted to them. Professional nursing, offered with a concept of nursing and high standards of professionalism, is awaiting its entry into these institutions, with which it shares a common goal—helping people.

chapter eight

Changes that have taken place

It is never easy to introduce change into a system crystallized by time and tradition. However, beginnings are being made through the thoughts and actions of professional nurses in several areas.

I salute, for example, the professional nurses in Wisconsin, and I hold them up as an example to be emulated whenever and wherever I speak or teach in the nation. They have brought about noteworthy changes in every setting—hospitals, clinics, nursing homes, juvenile delinquent homes, industry and community agencies. The professional nurses there have moved, on a sound intellectual basis, more rapidly and in larger numbers than nurses in any other state that I have visited in the presentation of new ideas. As I have told those nurses in Wisconsin who have effected change, I predict that nurses in other parts of the country will seek them out for assistance in initiating change in their own settings.

Special tribute must be paid to the late May Hornback, R.N., Ph.D., of the University of Wisconsin-Extension. She was prophetic in 1973, when she and I planned the course "Physical Assessment in a Nursing Frame of Reference." Dr. Hornback and I agreed so completely on the point that the "new knowledge" as presented in the literature was set in a medical frame of reference that we snatched up the opportunity to teach the content in a nursing frame of reference. The course was federally funded and has been continually refunded. There has always been a waiting list of applicants. I have taught the course 16 times (two days a month for three months), all over the state—in Madison, Eau Claire, Oshkosh, Superior and elsewhere. The visits to Wisconsin have been a highlight of my career, especially so in regard to the phase of independent practice. Because the courses have been offered in all parts of the state, there now exists a statewide awareness of the thinking of professional nurses concerning change in the field of nursing.

I would also like to recognize Miss Barbara Gessner of Wisconsin-Extension and Mrs. Shirley Berglund, independent nurse practitioner in the Minnesota Chemical Dependency Clinic, who assist in the laboratory sessions of my course. Mrs. Berglund's situation is an example of the change that is slowly taking place in various settings. She came to the course to help with the laboratory work, became interested in my ideas and says that as a result, she now practices independently at the Chemical Dependency Clinic, even though she works with two physicians. She says that they regard her as a colleague and adds, "I would be a physician's assistant if I hadn't come in contact with your ideas."

In addition, several of my Wisconsin students have reported changes that they have helped to bring about. In 1974, for example, professional nurses at St. Michael's Hospital in Stevens Point, Wisconsin, after taking my physical assessment course, formulated and presented a similar class to their staff nurses. "No rapid advances were made," said Donna Warzynski, R.N., "but subtle signs of spread of the concept to our peers became more and more evident each day. The data bases, patient assessments done on admission, became more meaningful and useful in meeting the needs of the client." When in 1975 drastic hiring restrictions and cutbacks threatened the quality of professional nursing care given at the hospital, the Nursing Service Management Team wrote a memorandum to the hospital administration underscoring the decline in quality of care and requesting changes to restore good care. As they aptly said, "You cannot dangle the opportunity to do professional nursing in front of us and keep moving it farther away from us each time we just barely touch it."

After that action, other nurses at the hospital began to take some positive steps themselves, Mrs. Warzynski said. "Because of various incidents with the medical staff and because these incidents compromised the time available for professional nursing, another letter was written by a group of professional nurses representing the Staff Nurse Organization." The letter read as follows:

> To the Medical Staff:
>
> At the January meeting of the Staff Nurse Organization growing concern was expressed by those present over an apparent communication barrier between doctors. It was felt that with increasing frequency a nurse is forced to play a role in which she is conveying vital information from one doctor to another, usually by phone. The reasons for this are not quite clear, but a number of actual situations described seemed to indicate that there is a convenience factor for the doctor or a hesitancy of one doctor to phone a colleague and speak to him directly. At those times, there seemed to exist a feeling of personal animosity between the physicians involved. Many times the exchange of information for which the nurse is then responsible becomes very sensitive, complex, conflicting, and time-consuming. We feel very vehemently that a nurse's first and foremost responsibility is to the patient, not to the doctor. Time spent on the phone transferring messages back and forth from one doctor to another, when the exchange of information could be done firsthand between the doctors involved, is time spent away from the patient. We do not exist for the convenience of the physician and object strongly to being caught in the middle of apparently differing opinions of how to practice medicine.
>
> At this same meeting, following our discussion of these communication problems, many nurses cited specific examples of situations that pointed up a grave problem of definition; i.e., how we define nursing as opposed to the physician's definition of a nurse. The fact that we are often

used as "sounding boards" for frustrated doctors is very discouraging and ill-taken. A physician's disagreements and problems with another
department of the hospital or with another doctor are not our concern unless we are used as
resources to help resolve those difficulties. We,
as professional nurses, are educated to be nursing practitioners, caregivers. We are able to
delineate between medical care and nursing
care. We do not give medical care; however, we
resent being denied the time and full rein to
give nursing care.
We are looking forward to working with you
as professional colleagues.

The Staff Nurse Organization

Mrs. Warzynski reports that the letter led to
a meeting with physicians in which the nurses were able to
present their philosophy of nursing and their view of the role
of the professional nurse in the hospital setting. "Clearly the
road is nowhere near complete," she says, "but I believe the
paving material is strong and will not crack under pressure."

And there are other changes. Two years ago
the hospital admission interview at St. Michael's was changed to
include information about the individual's health practices. According to June Page, R.N., interviews regarding health practices "are most beneficial in determining with the client his self-
care assets and deficits." And steps were taken to meet the client
needs expressed. For example, when the interviews revealed
that only one in ten women was doing breast self-examination
on a regular basis, the nurses began teaching the procedure to
interested women. "During our program we stress the normals
and knowing what is normal. We try to create healthy psychological attitudes." Miss Page says the reception given to this
self-care agency has been excellent.

Also at St. Michael's Hospital, a few months
ago problem-oriented charting was implemented in a 200-bed
acute care agency, and it was necessary for the nurses not only
to make assessments and plan for care, but also to document
those actions. The self-care concept was incorporated into the
new system. "As the nurses become more skilled in problem
identification, assessment and planning of care, it becomes evi-

dent that the client must become involved," said Marge Lund-
quist, R.N. "This involvement should focus on the client's assets
and his ability to mobilize these in managing his altered health
state. An example of this approach comes from a recent discussion by several of our professional nurses. Obesity had been
identified as a problem by the nurse admitting this patient for
abdominal surgery. In discussing her problem list with one of
her peers it became apparent that the other nurse disagreed
with her identifying obesity. She felt that the client might not
perceive himself as obese—so how could the nurse involve him?
'Coming from where the client is' seemed to be what this nurse
was saying. The plan was designed to include the patient in a
discussion of obesity and risk factors and then to move in the
direction he decided upon." This approach to managing alterations in a state of health and in practicing nursing in the hospital
setting is most promising.

"At this point," she continues, "our staff is
just into POR and it is difficult to determine what long-range
effects it will have on the practice of nursing. The biggest benefit that I see personally is the change in thinking on the part of
the professional nurse. She has become more aware of her
unique value to the client. She has had surprisingly little difficulty in identifying nursing problems, not medical problems.
She has enhanced her self-image by identifying the many facets
of care in which she is involved."

When I attended the second follow-up conference on the Wisconsin course in May, 1976, I asked the
nurses to send copies of material documenting changes they had
effected—such as those mentioned above—to the Center for
Nursing in Hattiesburg, Mississippi, so that this material could
be the point of departure for research projects there.

The Center for Nursing itself represents a
major change that will have repercussions in the entire field of
nursing. Located on the campus of the University of Southern
Mississippi, the Center opened in the fall of 1976, with three
major components—education, practice and research. The Center, under the deanship of Elizabeth Harkins, Ph.D., will serve
as an intellectual arena for nursing students, professional nurse
practitioners and nurse researchers. I am a visiting professor in

the School of Nursing and will coordinate the professional nursing care at the Center. One week every month I teach at the Center and see clients in my office there. My practice in Maryland served as the model for a practice affiliated with the Center for Nursing. When the Center is in full operation, students will be able to observe me giving nursing care to my clients (with the client's permission). This is a first in the history of nursing— the first professional nurse in independent practice has collaborated with the dean and faculty of a school of nursing to open the first Center for Nursing while continuing her private practices, in and out of state. The significance of the Center is that, for the first time, practice and education—with research in both areas—will be centralized. Every other profession has such centers, which serve as depositories for the major work being done in that particular profession. Until now nursing has had no such resources in a central location, and the establishment of the Center will make a big contribution toward helping the profession of nursing grow in stature.

One of the unique features of the Center for Nursing is that it offers to the post-master's degree nursing student the opportunity to study through a learnership. If accepted for this program, a nurse can study for a period ranging from one month to a year. The nurse pays her own expenses and chooses the length of time she wishes to study. The research conducted at the facility will be coordinated so that an objective can be identified and the steps needed to reach the goal spelled out in the overall design of the research. Master's students at the University of Southern Mississippi will contribute to the development of research projects as part of their degree requirements.

As the Center's brochure states, "The uniqueness of the Center for Nursing lies in the fact that there has never been such an institution. This will be the first time in history that nursing care will be offered to the public as a completely autonomous enterprise as evidenced by these factors in the total operation:

1. All aspects of the endeavor will be entirely controlled by professional nurses. The guidelines for organizational structure and policy of an academic nature are being developed

by the dean and the faculty of the School of Nursing of the University of Southern Mississippi.

2. As a first step in caring for their health, people can decide to make appointments with the professional nurse for nursing care.

3. This first step taken by the people themselves is contingent on one factor and one only, namely, their decision to seek professional nursing care.

4. There will be the establishment of a legitimate relationship between a professional person and the person seeking his services; this will be formally recognized in the rendering of a fee to the professional nurse.

5. The professional nurse will make judgments, initiate nursing care measures and be accountable to the client for the outcomes of these measures.

The pivotal points of the idea of this Center are basic ones which every professional practice discipline has as its sine qua non. In terms of its practice component, the points of departure are:

1. Availability through a recognized formal system, so that the public can avail itself of the service.

2. Accessibility to the professional person by an individual who may select the professional person he wants when he has a need for that professional care.

3. Accuracy of service rendered by the members of the professional practice discipline, with an integral plan for ongoing evaluation of the effectiveness of the care.

4. Accountability on a one-to-one basis to the persons served. Contact must be made between the professional person and the person whom he serves.

5. Autonomy of functioning by individuals in the profession, which assures the autonomy that a professional practice discipline must have.

In terms of the educational component of a professional practice discipline, the points of departure are:

1. The need for a service arena for students so that they can learn the practice from practitioners, which supplies the necessary dimension of learning the art of the profession as the science of the discipline is being implemented.

2. The need for the student to learn, with guidance from the teachers, the actual practice of the profession.

3. The need for the practitioner to study and upgrade his care on a continuing basis.

In terms of the research component of a professional practice discipline, the points of departure are:

1. As students learn nursing as it is practiced by other practitioners, and as they are practicing it themselves, areas for research become apparent.

2. The needs for research will emerge from an educational viewpoint as well as from a practice viewpoint.

3. The focus of professional nursing in the Center will generate hypotheses not heretofore tested in the practice of nursing.

4. Coordination of research as it progresses is essential because the effectiveness of the research in application prescinds from the cohesive nature of the overall research endeavors."

When several members of the graduate faculty were discussing the clinical experience for the students in the fall of 1975, the major problem identified was that the students were finding it difficult, in traditional settings, to apply the concept of nursing practice being taught at the University of Southern Mississippi. We agreed that a new type of facility was needed. Plans started to grow, and it was agreed that I would develop the idea, based on my own practice in Maryland. The individuals who planned the Center are Dean Elizabeth Harkins, Cora Balmat, Mary Colette Smith and Peggy Broomhall. The vision and foresight these nursing colleagues have shown in the development of the idea will be documented for history as the effect of the Center for Nursing is felt around the nation.

Changing attitudes are appearing farther to the east as well. At Georgetown University Hospital in Washington, D.C., professional nurses who practice within a concept of nursing and who can establish legitimate nurse-client relationships are available on one unit. When I gave a course to professional nurses at Georgetown, Mrs. Meriam Van Eron was one of my students. As a result of that course, Mrs. Van Eron was able to implement the plans she had been evolving for years. The various facets of her ideas blended with the content that I presented in the class, and she was able to move ahead with the initiation of changes on the units for which she was responsible. The integration of the notion of the professional aspect of the nursing care that patients receive on the Georgetown unit mentioned above has produced documented change in the care that the patients receive. This situation is a good example of the fact that the soundness of an idea is attested to when many people respond by identifying similarities between the speaker's thinking and position and their own viewpoint. On a continuing basis, I get this kind of response from the majority of my colleagues in nursing.

Last year the University of Virginia's School of Continuing Education asked me to teach the physical assessment course I taught at Wisconsin. The course was given to professional nurses in February, March and April, and the response was such that I was asked to teach it again in 1977. I would like to pay tribute to the vision of Mrs. Ann Lewis and Mrs. Betty Puzak, both professional nurses as well as faculty members in the School of Continuing Education.

It should be noted that the registrants for the courses in Wisconsin and Virginia represent diverse settings and varied training. In Wisconsin, the class was originally limited to those who deal directly with persons needing nursing care, a requirement that excluded educators and administrators. This was not the case in Virginia, because no federal monies were requested. In Virginia, therefore, the students were quite diverse. They included, for instance: a professional nurse with a Ph.D. who had taken a federally funded program for nurse practitioners; a nursing student; nurses with such titles as staff nurse, head nurse; supervisors; inactive nurses and teachers; public health nurses and nurses in industry. Despite the diversity, students in the class noted that everyone was discussing *nursing*, and that no one seemed threatened by the others as she presented her assignments regarding nursing care. In the past it has been difficult for persons from such diverse settings to find a common ground and discuss nursing without competition or defensiveness among the discussants. The message they received was the uniqueness of each professional nurse, free to give nursing care if proceeding from sound scientific bases and concepts, with judgments based on signals from the client that can be documented. The message was that a nurse is professional and responsible, and that a professional person can act independently.

Of course, there may be changes being implemented about which I have no knowledge, and I would appreciate hearing of them from my colleagues. I can only assume—and hope—that the more than 300 speeches I have given in recent years to groups throughout the country have stimulated new ways of thinking about nursing. This hope is based on comments that have been made to me after the speeches, comments such as: "After hearing you today, I know that my idea of nursing will never be the same."—"This will be the rebirth of nursing."—"I wish I had not heard you today because I know I will never be the same, that I have to go back and do something about it; and I know it's going to be hard."

I have no way of knowing how many of those persons and others in the audience have returned to their varied settings intending to implement changes. Even if my speeches have resulted only in changed attitudes that as yet remain latent, it is exciting to me to think that perhaps some day, in some way, those attitudes will come to the fore and provide the impetus for the transformation of professional nursing.

The actions described in this chapter represent significant starting points for that transformation. But there is still so much work to be done. I call on professional nurses everywhere to help us continue.

APPENDIX:
Client examples

Throughout the years of my practice I have always wanted to talk about my clients and the nursing care that I have given them. When the time came for me to sit down at the typewriter and write about them for this book, I found myself in a terrible dilemma. When I condensed the material about a specific client, even I could not recognize the person for whom I had cared. When I enlarged upon it in an effort to make the person and his needs come alive for the reader and to show how I had exercised my judgment in regard to his self-care assets and deficits and his therapeutic self-care demands, the narration called for such detail that it became tedious to write and even more tedious to read. The problem is clearly this: the mind-set of the reader of this material will correspond to the concept of "nurse" and "nursing" that he or she holds. This will be true whether the reader is a lay person or a nurse. Whether the material is abridged or detailed, the essence of nursing in my practice lies in the thought processes that I engaged in as I pursued a course of action in regard to a particular client's needs. And to be able to recount those thought processes fully, it would have been necessary for me to have recorded them as they progressed during the client session. To have done so, to have paid such close attention to my thoughts as they developed, would have diffused the attention I had to focus on the expressions of need—verbal and nonverbal—emanating from the client, and would consequently have weakened the nursing care being given. Indeed, to hang upon every word of the client—which the professional nurse must do if she is to hear what is being communicated to her—and simultaneously to hang upon every thought of my own would be a monumental task. However, it is a task which clearly must be accomplished in professional nursing. This situation is another striking example of the need for nursing research and documentation. During my early years as a professional independent nurse, what was happening between me and my clients was so new that at the time even I would not have been able to describe it fully to myself or others. To be able to do so remains yet another challenge of my nursing career.

In addition to that problem, one of the main difficulties is that I am dealing with material the significance of which I do not yet fully comprehend myself. It is similar to any research study in which the data have been gathered and have yet to be analyzed—or, as in this case, the experimentation has been done (establishing an independent nursing practice), but all of the data have yet to be fully recorded.

For example, I have classified as primarily supportive and secondarily therapeutic that nursing care which I give in the first four phases of the health history described in Chapter 4. I have to give nursing care to help the client express his nursing needs. That nursing action has to be analyzed in detail to identify "what I did for that person, for that client." In the fifth and sixth phases the care that I give is primarily therapeutic and secondarily supportive.

At this point in my experience, I can determine to a fair degree of accuracy the way in which the client will verbalize his needs. I have classified characteristics of expression of need by the client, and it is important to recognize the differences, because the nursing care should be varied according to the way in which the client expresses his needs. This becomes tangible only after many cases are studied.

It is essential to sound a cautionary note as professional nurses begin to read about the clients. The tendency in the nursing world to label makes it necessary to point out that the approach I use in giving nursing care to my clients is different from the traditional way of categorizing nursing needs. For example, when I have told some nurses about my clients, the response has been, "Oh, that is a psychological need," or, "That is an emotional need," or, "That is a geriatric need." I simply cannot think of the needs of my clients in that way. As the client examples will show, the nursing approach has been to recognize and incorporate the body, mind and spirit of the person in a way that has not been done before in the recognition of needs, the definition of self-care assets and deficits and the construction of nursing measures. Depending on the direction that the client indicates he wishes to take, the physical aspect is often secondary in the nursing situation (and is often being dealt with medically by a physician), whereas the needs of mind and spirit are primary.

At the risk of sounding self-aggrandizing, I must tell the readers how I feel about the nursing care that I give. In the worlds of music and art, there are limits to what the artists can do. The limits are in the form of the canvas, the pallette, the colors, the instrument, the hands. The picture in the mind of the artist demands to be expressed, to be communicated to others. In law, the limits are the facts. What the lawyer does with them becomes the art of the practice of law. In my practice, the limits are the concept within which I practice and the needs expressed by my clients. I too wish to transmit to others the picture that is in my mind as I give care to my clients. The fault lies in the inadequacies of the written and spoken word.

The reader may find it helpful to approach the reading of the client examples by this process:

1. Try to erase all previous experiences from the mind. Read the words, but do not manipulate them.
2. Do not try to interpret the interaction between the nurse and the client.

3. Do not try to fill in the points that would make the situation seem familiar to you.

4. If it seems so familiar to you that you find yourself asking the question, "What is new about this?" then ask yourself the question, "Am I taking an action carried out by the nurse out of the concept of professional nursing practice?" If the answer is "no," then I ask you the question, "What is *your* concept of professional nursing practice?"

       It must also be remembered by the reader that the client examples are simplified synopses of specific client sessions or sequences of sessions, and that the actual nursing process is continuous and evolutionary over a period of weeks or years. In this section, I will briefly describe a situation and then outline some of the self-care assets and deficits involved, as well as some nursing measures. Although the reader may not be able to see in detail the complexity of the nursing situation, it is hoped that this material, in addition to the client examples given in other chapters, will provide some idea of the kind (and scope) of needs for which people seek professional nursing care. In two examples, I have copied the sheets from my notebook so that an idea of the intricacy of the action involved in making a nursing judgment may be gleaned. The dynamic flow is extremely hard to recapitulate; yet it is this characteristic of client contact that is the essence of nursing care. As a result of the initial analysis of data gathered in researching the making of judgments by a professional nurse, I have identified the characteristics of expression of need by the client. The demand for a high degree of skill in making judgments is obvious when one realizes that the essence of making a professional nursing judgment consists in the assimilation of the variety of nursing needs expressed by the individual client and the weighing of several aspects simultaneously. The skill with which supportive nursing care is given will produce an accurate recounting of need by the clients, and this in turn will result in more effective therapeutic nursing care—which also requires skill in conveying its intent to the client.

Characteristics of expression of need by the client

These characteristics have been identified after five years of practice:

Key: Need is represented by V

1. Some clients express their needs very directly. They will say, "My need is. . . ," or "I made an appointment with you because. . . ." Many times the verbalized need is intricately bound up with a larger need, and the relationship is significant. This is referred to as a *narrowed* need.

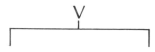

2. Some clients express their needs in a global manner, and the most pressing need may not emerge for a period of time. The immediate need may be encompassed by larger needs, and the relationship is significant. This is referred to as an *encompassed* need.

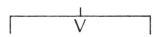

3. Some clients express their needs in a labyrinthine fashion. The mode of expression is significant as an indication of the nature of the client's need. This is referred to as a *segmented* need.

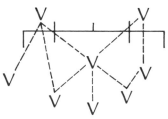

IMPLICATIONS: Identification of complexity of nursing needs which will be highly important in curriculum development.

Client example 1

"I would like you to be my professional nurse. Can I make an appointment to see you? I want to talk over some things that are distressing me. I want to ask you some questions to see if I have the right perspective."

The client, a practical nurse, was 24 years old when she first contacted me. During our client sessions, she would tell me about the interactions she was having with the person for whom she is caring and with that person's family. "Miss Kinlein," she would say, "You always speak the truth, and that means so much to me. Now tell me whether I did something I should have done or something I should not have done." Then she would describe the situation to me. Frequently, the situation involved several personalities, as well as her care of an elderly lady (also a client of mine) and her own goals in life. Later the client had medical needs, which were also a consideration in the nursing care she received.

Working with the client with regard to the way she cared for the elderly person was important to her total health state. The client is incapable of tolerating less than optimum standards for the care of people, and she maintains this level of care through sheer self-discipline, on a daily basis—for 24 hours when she is alone with the person under her care. In her view of herself as a nurse, she placed a high value on self-discipline and insisted on upholding her standards—attitudes that are reflected in her ambitious and scrupulous care of people. The way I work with her as my client demands the integration of her values for herself as a person and as a nurse.

One of the problems confronting my client was the misrepresentation of her care of the elderly woman by a family friend, who fostered misunderstanding between the woman and her family and cast suspicion on my client's daily management of the environment of nursing care. In dealing with this situation, the client's self-care assets included a desire to be an active participant in bringing about change that would reestablish her sense of inner peace and harmony and her ability to retain dignity and a sense of integrity throughout all encounters. She also had an acute awareness of the value of patience and long-suffering in her total set of values. Self-care deficits included her inability to control her emotions at times and to articulate her own position in the heat of confrontation; the assistance she needed in coping with the assault on her pride; and her nonrecognition of her real contribution to the care of the elderly person. The therapeutic self-care demand after the first appointment was the need for the client to focus attention on her own set of values, in order to gain a perspective on her reactions and responses to the series of events that faced her daily. The nursing care measures consisted of proposals made by me for the client's consideration and choice, after I had put forth the specific benefits to be expected from each course of action, as well as the possible negative results.

At the agreement of my client, the nursing care measure followed involved my meeting with the family friend concerned, as well as another meeting between the family friend and my client. After I had received information from both my client and the family friend about the situation, the nursing intervention I designed included laying the facts before both, setting ground rules for discussion of the facts and pointing out digressions from the issue under consideration at the moment. My client became relaxed as the discussion proceeded, and the other person failed to see the validity of some of my client's opinions and comments. My client, in turn, was able to recognize when her words and actions were the result of motivation that was not in accordance with the fundamental tenets by which she lives. (The effectiveness of this line of nursing judgment and action depends on having the verbalized feelings and positions of the client as data on which to act.)

Several such meetings were held and my client's health state improved. She reported that she began to enjoy her food more; she became relaxed and was able to sleep more. The persistent nausea from which she had been suffering decreased, as did the amount of gas in her intestinal tract and the slight discomfort in her stomach, which she said sometimes became painful.

There were several appointments in the next year. In assessing the total nursing care she received the client said, "You gave me a sense of my own worth and importance. I have so much more confidence in myself, and that is because you helped me to see all my strengths. I used to be quiet in any group. I enjoyed being with people, but I never used to say much. Now I have the security of feeling that I can say something and people will listen to me."

Two years after the initial contact with this client, gastric discomfort exacerbated. The medical diagnosis was hiatal hernia and duodenitis, and the treatment was Valium and an antacid. The pain subsided. In a few months the client reported pain in another area of the body and major surgery was indicated for removal of uterine tumors, which were benign. She made a most unusual recovery from the operation, with no complications and no pain, except for the night following surgery, and she regained her physical strength very rapidly. Her mental state was excellent throughout the whole period of diagnosis, treatment and follow-up care. She attributes her rapid recovery to the professional nursing care she received before, during and after the surgical period.

Client example 2

Another client, who has been receiving my nursing care for four years, is a 36-year-old woman who opened her discussion of her health state with this prefatory comment: "I don't want to be treated like a two-year-old." She had recently had open heart surgery at a large teaching hospital; she expressed distaste about the way she had been treated and was still upset by it. My first contact with her told me that she had a great deal of self-respect and pride and that she was a religious woman. She reported that the episode began with severe pain in her ankle. When she went for diagnosis of the problem, she was told that she needed heart surgery. Her ankle was not treated, and she continued to complain of constant pain in her ankle. Over and over again, she would tell me about her hospital experience and about the fact that the tone of voice used by the physicians and nurses was like that used in addressing children. "You don't talk to a mature woman as though she didn't have the ability to understand what you are saying to her."

During the second or third appointment she asked me about the nature of the surgery that had been performed on her heart. She showed me the hospital form that accompanied the bill and asked about some of the tests that had been performed. Since she had been employed in a nursing home, she was looking forward to returning to gainful employment, but the medical opinion was that she could not go back to work for about six months. She took a typing course after a social worker and I had had several conferences with her, but she was unable to pass the typing tests. Other attempts to help her obtain employment were unsuccessful. She was on welfare because of her medical disability and has never been able to work since her heart surgery.

On every house call she complained about the pain in her ankle, which was largely ignored by the physicians. Her physical condition deteriorated. She began to eat more and more and gained much weight. Finally she went to an orthopedic specialist, who prescribed a special kind of shoe, but no relief was provided. She was operated on finally for the degeneration of the ankle bone and since then her ankle has not bothered her. However, she was told that she had arthritis of the hip and that she should have surgery for it. I asked her if her hip had ever bothered her. "No, it has not bothered me," she said, "but the doctor said that I need to have it done." Since the hip surgery she has had constant, intense pain in her hip and walks with a limp. She has had to have more and more medication to relieve the pain and help her sleep. She has had additional heart surgery, following which she experienced multiple complications. She stayed in the hospital for two months and is now in a rehabilitation hospital. Her needs are so great that they would keep a professional nurse busy 24 hours a day.

Throughout the nursing care sessions that she requested, some of the self-care assets that emerged were patience acquired through many situations that degraded her as a human being, a strong sense of self-respect and pride, religious faith, and the ability to understand complex situations when the professional person approached her with respect. The self-care deficits were her inability to sustain hope and to avoid despair and her inability to alter the need for medication. Some nursing care measures were to have her focus on and list her abilities, in an effort to maintain her sense of worth; to continue to have faith in God and to continue to seek clarification of her medical condition and to recognize that she can decide, after being given the necessary facts, whether or not to have the medical treatment prescribed.

The nursing care centered on providing support for her in keeping a viable self-image in light of all that continues to happen to her. She says she relies on my nursing care and could not have gotten through her problems without it. Medically, the client has had so many complications following the open heart surgery that her return to her home cannot at this point be predicted.

Client example 3

A 26-year-old woman came to me with a request for blood work, a CBC, because she wanted information about her hemoglobin count. She described her feeling of fatigue and the intense pain in her joints. She decided to see a specialist in arthritis. The medical diagnosis was neuromuscular disorder of unknown etiology. The pain persisted. One day she told me she thought she was pregnant, which was later confirmed. About six weeks later she had to enter the hospital because of dehydration caused by excessive vomiting. She had also experienced an episode of fainting. Throughout the remainder of her pregnancy she was healthy, she was attractive in physical appearance and had a positive mental attitude. The father of her child was delighted with the pregnancy, and the home environment was tranquil and happy. She delivered a boy (weight 9 lb 6 oz) and was elated that the baby was healthy. Two days after delivery, however, she had convulsions, fell, broke a front tooth, and had to undergo diagnostic tests. She developed paralysis of her right side because of the pressure of a blood clot on the brain. Surgery was performed and for several days her life was in danger. After a month in the hospital she went to stay with her parents. Her physical appearance had changed drastically because of the shaving of her waist-length hair, the chipped tooth, her wanness and occasional strabismus. There was family tension, with pressure regarding her unmarried status and stress generated by the child's father because she and the baby were not at home with him. Through sheer determination she recovered the use of her right side and gained enough strength to take the baby back to their apartment.

The situation was such that she would contact me and express an acute need following an argument with the child's father, or an argument or misunderstanding with her parents. At the same time, she had to cope with numerous and difficult arrangements for her medical care. For example, she had to have hearing tests in conjunction with assessing the brain trauma. The physician told her to return so that he could tell her about the results. She made the appointment a month in advance. On the day of the appointment her father took time off from work to drive her 35 miles to the hospital to see the physician. There was an empty waiting room, but she waited 30 minutes without the receptionist's saying a word to her. When she inquired about the delay, the response was, "We can't call the doctor until your chart comes." "But," the client said, "the appointment was made a month ago. I'm very tired, but I'll wait another ten minutes." In ten minutes the chart still had not arrived. The client told the receptionist she was going to leave, and the receptionist said, "But you have to stay to talk to the doctor to know the results of the test." The client decided to leave anyway, because at the time the tests were made the technician had told her the results looked very good. Such situations, which were numerous throughout her difficulties, complicated the client's problems and made coping with them that much harder.

Medically, when the client was discharged after hospitalization for convulsions, a definitive diagnosis regarding the cause of the convulsions was still lacking. However, she was classified as epileptic and Dilantin and phenobarbital therapy was prescribed. Because of these medical uncertainties, the client became concerned and began making plans for a will, to establish custody of her child. The financial aspect of the lives of mother, father and son is bleak—the hospital bill is $9,000, they have difficulty making their rent payments, and the telephone had to be disconnected.

Throughout her nursing care, the self-care assets at work for the client were her inner strength, which enabled her to survive enormously stressful situations, her love of nature, her belief in people and her great capability to love. Her biggest self-care deficits were the inability to modify her environment so that serenity could be achieved and indecision regarding her relationship with the father of her child. Nursing care measures included helping her to decide to contact a physician about the pain in her joints, establishing criteria for judging how she felt about the child's father and whether or not to remain with him, and helping her to understand her part in reestablishing good relations with her family. Nursing care measures are also taken on behalf of the baby. For example, I take the child and his mother to the clinic for the baby's immunization shots and remain with them. The mother tells her friends that she would not have been able to get through so much adversity had it not been for the nursing care she receives and she boasts that her son is my client, too. That this client has remained intact through so many difficult situations is indeed remarkable.

Client example 4

A woman brought her one-and-a-half-year-old daughter to me for a nursing evaluation of the child's paralyzed left arm and left leg. She told me that a physician had told her to wait until the child was five to begin therapy. Based upon knowledge of the child's condition from the health history and of the nature of contracted muscles, my suggestion was that therapy should begin now. With the agreement of the child's mother, I established passive exercises with her and outlined a plan of attaching progressively heavy weights to the arm after the muscle had been relaxed through exercises, thus pulling the arm down into an extended position. The child's mother engaged her babysitter in the project and in several months the change in the extremities was dramatic. Nursing care continued after the orthopedist devised lightweight arm braces for the child to wear while sleeping and a light brace that is attached to her shoe while she walks during the day. The child's mother also has made appointments with me for herself, when she has had questions about her health state, and she comes to me for physical examinations.

The self-care assets at work in this situation were the mother's knowledge that care was needed for the child, her marked ability to implement nursing measures, and her exercise of good judgment about modifications of therapeutic measures. The self-care deficit was the need for verification of her perceptions of the child's needs and progress. The outcome has been a dramatic improvement in the use of the child's arm and leg. The care that I gave to the father, mother and child was a point of reference for them in their decision-making about the medical needs of the child.

Client example 5

I received a call at home one morning from the husband of a client I have had for four years. He said that his wife had fallen in the night and had cut her forehead. He had tried to stop the bleeding, but it was continuing. He asked if I could come over to see his wife.

When I arrived the client's face was streaked with dried and fresh blood, and blood was running through her hair over her ear, so that for the period of inspection of the total picture, I was not sure if she had suffered a skull fracture or additional injury to the cut on her head, which was a laceration about two inches long. I washed her face, ears and neck with soap and water while her husband went to the drugstore for hydrogen peroxide, adhesive tape and four-by-four gauze squares. I used full-strength hydrogen peroxide to irrigate the wound and then made butterflies to approximate the edges of the wound. Later, the husband called and said that there had been no more bleeding, not even the oozing of serum which I had said might drain for a while. The physical examination revealed no other injuries, and no symptoms of skull fracture or concussion appeared. Subsequently, the scar was almost imperceptible.

A major factor in my decision-making about the condition of the woman was the long-standing relationship I had with her and her husband and, in particular, my experience with the husband on previous occasions when it had been necessary that he describe something to me. I had always found his awareness of the importance of details supplied to me a solid basis for my proceeding along a particular path. In the last six months, for example, in caring for his wife he has carried out the measurement of fluid intake and output with greater accuracy than I have seen in many hospital situations.

This example represents only one episode in the continuous nursing care I have given this couple in helping them meet their needs in light of the wife's illness, Huntington's chorea. The self-care assets to draw upon are the marked degree of love between the husband and wife, acceptance of the facts of the wife's illness, the husband's inventiveness in regard to cooking and caring for his wife, and the husband's recognition that he must stay alert in order to meet his wife's needs. The self-care deficits include the need to combine a satisfactory work schedule with the care schedule for his wife and the need for support in coping with small and large problems in the wife's care. Nursing care measures have been for the clients to recognize the reserve of strength they possess in the love they have for each other and to establish and maintain a routine of care. The outcome has been that a degree of stability and serenity has been achieved by both.

Client example 6

A similar client need arose with a 95-year-old man for whom I had been caring for a number of years. His daughter had engaged my services in the care of her father, and I had been giving him a bath weekly for a year. One morning she called me and said that her father had fallen and cut his head. Would I come over to look at it? Examination of the posterior bony prominence of the skull revealed a right angle skin laceration with an uneven smaller cut extending from the angle itself. I washed the wound with peroxide, cut some hair away, approximated the edges with a sterilized tweezer and smoothed out the skin. I put merthiolate on the cut and applied a small loose bandage to be removed in two days. It healed without complications.

I continued to care for the client weekly. One afternoon after I had just arrived and taken off my coat, the client's daughter and I heard a thump. We went to the hallway, where we found the client lying prone. Apparently he had wrapped himself in a blanket when he was getting ready for his bath and had tripped over the edge of the blanket when he started to walk. His shoulder struck the wall with great force, and when I examined him I found that his shoulder was fractured. His daughter and I staved off clinical shock and tried to keep edema to a minimum while we waited for a medical transportation service to take him to the hospital. The nursing care given during that time was designed to reduce the client's fear and to support his need to maintain dignity and control. This was accomplished, and in good time the ambulance arrived and took the client to the hospital.

In this situation the self-care assets included the client's sense of pride and independence, the daughter's sense of devotion to her father and her ability to make good judgments about his care, the daughter's willingness to try new measures for herself and her father, and the efforts of both to be self-sufficient in maintaining their care. The deficits are the client's physical inability to do things for himself and the need for help in coping on a day-to-day basis with both the daughter's and father's needs. Nursing care measures included their accepting that the need for help is a basic human need during life and trusting the judgments the daughter made in regard to her father and herself. On a weekly basis my nursing care was integrated by them into their regimen of health maintenance.

The father eventually died in a nursing home, and I assisted the daughter through her feelings of guilt and remorse. She continues to come for my nursing care in regard to losing weight and maintaining a good health state.

Client example 7

A 19-year-old college student made an appointment to see me one day. "I have been listening to your teaching about your nursing care, and I like your approach and the way you help people," he said. "I would like to have you help me with my problems. . . . I really don't know how to express my needs. . . . I have been feeling depressed. . . . I sleep a lot. . . . I am tired lately. . . . I don't know if it is physical or mental. . . . I have tremors which usually lead to crying. . . . It seems like every day I want to get over it, and every day it comes back. Whenever I feel mixed up, I always take a long walk, look at nature, and that helps a lot."

Through a series of sessions with this client, I helped him to identify his problems and established nursing care measures for each problem after a priority had been determined. The movement of my approach in nursing care was a global one initially, then a narrowing down of a particularly plaguing part of the problem that bothered him at that time, then a pulling back to get that progress in perspective, then a return to a more global approach, until finally he had a panoramic view of himself as a person, a student, a man, a son, and a Catholic.

On the first appointment his skin was broken out, his eyes were dull, his color sallow, his posture slumped and his voice level almost inaudible. His handshake was limp and he was tense. After the initial communication from him, I said, "Let's look at your self-care assets as I have picked them up as you spoke. First of all, you came to see me; you made an appointment to get help. Then you mentioned that you had a way of handling your mixed-up emotions—by taking long walks, being with nature, and that is helpful when some people feel the need to close out the rest of the world and get a handle on things. So you are able to take action at the time you feel mixed-up. That is a definite self-care asset. It would seem that a self-care deficit would revolve around the need to find additional measures to eliminate 'it.' (When I had asked him earlier to explain what he meant by 'it,' he had replied, "I guess I mean my outlook on life . . . that it's not going to get better.") We talked about his sensitivity as an asset, and he added that he didn't feel he could handle things or that he had self-confidence. "I don't know who I am. Feelings about myself change. Sometimes I think I know, and I can do things, and then other times I get all mixed-up. I seem to be all apart."

I responded, "One of the points that I would like to bring out to you is the evidence that I have of your self-discipline. You did something that required a certain togetherness of self, asking me for an appointment. There had to be insight to a degree in order to act on your conviction that you need help. Another instance is in regard to physical discipline—the way you take action in long walks. If we analyze your thinking processes and emotional processes step by step, it is possible to gain an adjusted viewpoint of what makes you *you*, and, through an evolutionary approach, to pinpoint areas that need concentrated focus. A gradual unfolding of the characteristics of your personality would seem to be an appropriate first step to take. How does that sound to you?" One of the nursing care measures instituted at this point was his keeping a diary listing the decisions he makes daily about big and little things.

On the second appointment he said he felt better. "I wrote down some decisions. That helped. The problem of getting up in the morning and living has to be worked at. When you talked with me last week about being patient with myself, that helped a lot, and I kept telling myself that all week. I have taken a lot better notes this last week. Sometimes I drift off and start to doodle. I bought a charcoal pencil and pad and thought, 'If I'm going to draw—I'll learn how to draw better.' Also, I thought a lot about nature, looked at nature and saw things created the way they are—right or wrong, good or bad. . . ." A program of sensible eating and sleeping was discussed and worked out, as well as various exercises, and the continued pursuit of solitude was encouraged.

During the third appointment he reported that he had a "very nice week—worked out better than ever. Your advice to trust my decisions was very good. Woke up not feeling too good, but there was no deep depression." He related a significant incident: "I was working on a film last night and I was messing up the splicing. Ordinarily, I would have persisted, but I thought it over and decided to go to bed." We discussed that decision as a first level of control. "If self-confidence is being shaken, stop for a short time; or, in this case, because of the hour, it was best to go to bed. The virtue of prudence was observed and demands both strength and restraint, action and inaction. Later on, the second level of control will be achievable—to persist, but the persistence will be preceded by careful analysis, relaxation, and then renewed concentration. For your age, your physical state, psychological state and hormonal state, you made the right decision. Conversely, this kind of decision *not* to do something under certain circumstances will build self-confidence in terms of what you can do."

By the fourth appointment he said, "I had several times this week when I didn't feel too good, but I was always able to pull myself out. In calming down, I think of what you told me: First, when I feel physically warm, I go out and take a walk, if I can. If I'm in a room, I stop, take a deep breath, relax, and the answer comes. I'm getting better at following through in regard to the class schedule. . . ." On a subsequent appointment he related that when he felt confused he would "do some work and calm down. I felt better." We discussed the relationship between physical action and the output of hormones in a teen-aged male.

I worked with this client using tools such as a diary, his sketches during and outside of class, and graphs of the stages in his improvement in regard to his "problems." (Examples follow.) The science of physiology was drawn on as I reached judgments about his physical and mental development, and my own strong philosophical views were a point of departure for him in developing his own philosophy about himself and his unique role in life. Among his self-care assets are an unusual degree of insight and perception into his needs and his ability to implement nursing care measures. His major self-care deficits were a lack of confidence that he could bring about changes, his feelings that he was different from other fellows and that he was never going to be able to mix well with groups of people.

Now, this client walks briskly, with his head up. His complexion is rosier, his handshake firmer. He speaks in a louder tone and smiles broadly. He says people have commented on the change in his appearance. He feels better inside himself, even though he still has difficult days.

EXPLANATION OF CHARTS

I drew up two charts, or graphs, to help my client understand his improvement in the various areas of self-care deficits that he had. I showed him his self-care assets, also, and indicated how he had continued to use these most effectively. The numbers are arbitrary ones, and the movement traced by the lines was an attempt on my part to help my client see the flow of his progress over a period of time. This is a graphic illustration of the professional appraisal that I made in the case of this particular client. I used this method because of his feeling of discouragement at the fact that he was not always continuing in the same progressive pattern, but would go forward and then backward in his outlook. The periods of regression were disturbing to him until he saw the steady improvement over all. (See charts on pages 155 and 156.)

Client example 8

Another client sought my nursing care because, as she put it, "I need support, I guess. I have reasoned out some things about myself, and I'd like to have you tell me whether or not I'm on the right track." The woman had had a diagnosis of congestive heart failure for a period of ten years. Her cardiologist had told her to make twice-a-year appointments to see him. When the client came to see me she had seen the physician six weeks previously, and he had said everything was all right. But the client said she felt she was going downhill, that her heart condition had changed, even though the tests were negative. She said she noticed she was retaining more fluid than usual. She felt fatigued. She wondered if she should go back to the doctor before the next scheduled appointment. I suggested checking her heart action through EKGs and recommended blood tests regarding the yellowish tint of her skin. The

SITUATIONS

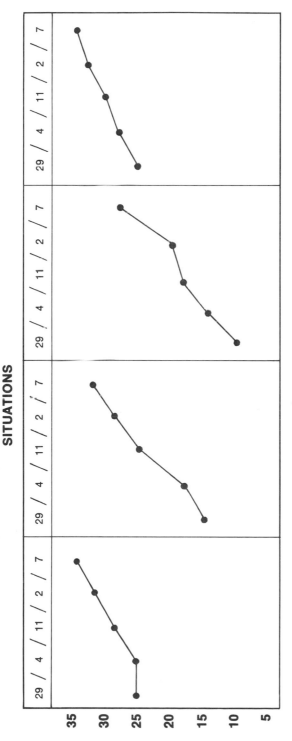

Analysis of Client's Progress—A

S-C Assets: (1) Initiate action on own
a) taking walks
b) exercise
c) helping parents
d) studying

(2) Control over self
a) set limits—movie
b) persevere with difficulty
in making decisions
c) getting up in A.M.

(3) Insight (developing)
a) friends
b) whole—not a part—clock
man
c) need to pull energy and
talent together
d) crying and urinating

(4) Ability to follow through
a) keeping notebook
b) measuring own progress
c) carrying out
assignments
d) "calm down," "forge
ahead," "follow my nose"

SITUATIONS

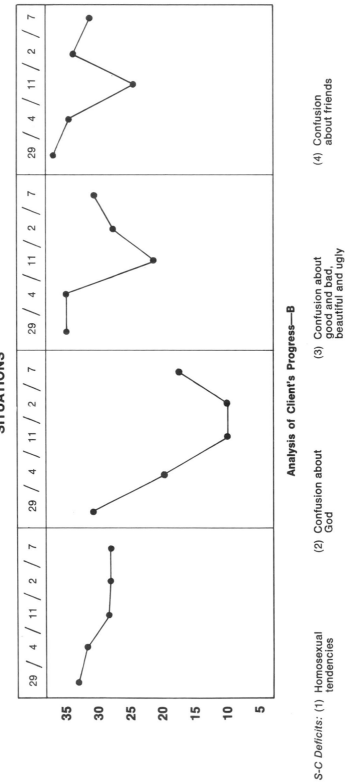

Analysis of Client's Progress—B

S-C *Deficits:* (1) Homosexual tendencies   (2) Confusion about God   (3) Confusion about good and bad, beautiful and ugly   (4) Confusion about friends

tests showed changes. She said she felt different from the way she had felt during previous illnesses caused by heart pathology, and nursing care helped her to decide to return to the cardiologist. She was subsequently hospitalized.

She asked me to make a hospital call and told me that one physician had diagnosed her condition as congestive heart failure and another had diagnosed cancer of the liver. "How could there be such different views? Aren't my symptoms definitive enough? Look at my abdomen with all that fluid." I drew a picture for her to explain the interference to the circulation in the liver that a deficient heart muscle could cause and that cancer of the liver could cause, with the result of ascites in both instances. She said, "You always make things clear for me, Miss Kinlein." She asked some more questions and then, after reflection, said, "You know what I think it is? I think it is cancer." I supported her thinking the situation out as she had done.

In the months that followed, after a final diagnosis of cancer, I made house calls, bathed her, stayed with her and answered her questions. One night she asked, "Will the radiation therapy make me better, Miss Kinlein?" I answered very gently that it would not. "I see. . . . The doctors keep saying, 'Try it for a few more weeks; it might make you feel better,' . . . but I know that each day I tell myself it can't be any worse tomorrow, but each tomorrow is worse. I would not be wrong to say I don't want any more treatments, would I? I would have tried long enough. . . . I have decided. I will tell the doctors that I will not take any more treatments." Then, after a long pause, she asked, "How will I react with no more treatments? I mean, will I be in excruciating pain? Will I lose consciousness? What is the usual progression of events in cases like mine?" After I explained the various possibilities, very gently, slowly, honestly, she said, "No matter what condition I'm in, please come for the appointments, because I will know you are here, even if I can't talk, if I'm in a coma. . . . The following week she was able to whisper only, "Dear Miss Kinlein, dear Miss Kinlein. . . ." After I left, the priest came, and she died two hours later.

The self-care assets in this situation were the client's knowledge of her physical state and her interpretation of the significance of change, the ability to work through a problem to a wise conclusion, and the acceptance of death. The deficits were an inability to care for herself, the inability to make a decision to change medical therapy. The nursing care measures she employed were to recall the good judgments made in the past about her health state and to trust her judgment now. The outcome was a peaceful death at home.

Client example 9

One nursing situation centered around a 23-year-old man who had taken mind-expanding drugs when he was in his teens, but has not taken any for the last two years. I gave nursing care to his parents regarding the transfer of their son from one institution to another. In every instance, the care he received was from a psychiatrist, either during private sessions or in group therapy. He had improved to the point where he had a job in a florist's shop. However, one day he left the area and his parents were notified that he was in another state. He was picked up by the police because he could not give an adequate explanation of why he was in the parking lot of a shopping center with a stolen credit card in his possession. When the parents contacted me, it was to ask for assistance in finding a facility for their son that was not like the controlled environment of a psychiatric institution. They wanted a facility that offered more freedom, because their son was able to understand that he needed care, but not the strict kind he received at the psychiatric institutions. I immediately started to make phone calls to get the information they had requested, because they were driving up to get their son that day, and the mother had said, "This is an S.O.S." As it turned out, there are no facilities of the kind the parents and I envisioned for the care of their son.

The parents said they would like me to meet their son and make a nursing assessment of his health state. They proposed the idea to their son and he agreed. As a result of the first house call I made, I recommended to the young man that he consider having nursing care on an intensive basis and suggested that in light of his needs, continuing contact with professional nurses who had studied in the area of mental health would supply the skills and expertise that I lacked. I suggested that he go for a month to Hattiesburg, Mississippi, for nursing at the Center for Nursing.

The client's self-care assets were his incisiveness in regard to his needs; an awareness of the effect of the medication given to him to relieve his depression—medication that made him callous to situations rather than helped him adjust to them; and honesty about his need for help, evident in all phases of interaction during the appointment. His self-care deficits were his inability to get a handle on his feelings so that he could take constructive action, his inability to apply his marked degree of intelligence to a given issue for a prolonged period of time, and his lack of awareness that he was in almost all respects 90 percent normal and that his behavior was within normal limits.

Nursing care measures were to remain concerned about himself because he felt as though he was trying to get better—and this awareness of self is good; to consider going to Mississippi for nursing care; and to concentrate on his feelings, thoughts and reactions that were well within normal limits. After the first appointment, he took the first bath he had taken in two weeks. After the second appointment he said he did not want to see me again, but as I was leaving he asked for my card "with a telephone number."

The care of this client marked the first time that I recommended care that can be obtained at the Center for Nursing in Hattiesburg, Mississippi. This kind of nursing care was not available before the opening of this facility. If the client decides to go there for nursing care, I will be his professional nurse and will engage the consulting services of nurses with expertise in the areas in which the client expresses a need. His activities will be controlled in conjunction with his exercise of self-care agency, and contacts at all hours of the day will be integrated into a plan of care that will approximate an average day in his life.

Client example 10

Another client came to me five years ago because she had questions about her health state. She had a history of Ménière's syndrome and had extreme shock reaction to drugs of all kinds. She has a very thorough understanding of herself and her metabolism, is aware of the aging process, and investigates new avenues of care in a suitably inquiring way. Two major episodes in the last year had given her concern. The first occurred when she choked on a piece of food and had to be taken to the emergency room because of extreme weakness following the choking spell and dislodgement of the food particle. She said she felt very close to death at that time and wanted to talk about it at one of our appointments.

The second episode occurred when an extremely severe attack of Ménière's syndrome incapacitated her to the point where she thought she might have to be hospitalized. She called around midnight and in an urgent, pleading voice begged me to be at the hospital so that no one would give her medication of any kind. She was crying for fear that the doctors and nurses at the hospital would not listen to her and was panicked at the prospect of a repetition of an extremely critical situation that had arisen when she could not convince physicians of her allergic reactions to the most commonly used drugs. I assured her, "I shall be there," in as definitive a tone as possible. "I will not let them give you any drug." I kept repeating that to her. She called back about 1:30 A.M. and again at 2:15 A.M. when the attack was beginning to subside. At 7 A.M. she said she felt much better, though very weak.

Throughout all of her health situations, this client's self-care assets were a knowledge of her own metabolism, an interest in new and valid methods of therapy, and her ability to take action even when under extreme pressure. The deficits were her inability to control events in the medical system and her physical debility. The nursing care measures were the knowledge that I would prevent the administration of medication that would lead to a crisis, and a continuation of the measures already initiated by the client in regard to the diarrhea accompanying the attack. The outcome was recovery from the episode at home.

Client example 11

One client engaged my nursing care when she was facing surgery for removal of a cataract in her left eye.

She was extremely anxious and apprehensive and would make an appointment for a house call when she had a sore throat, or when she thought her blood pressure was up. She broke a tooth and was sure that she could not have the surgery because of it. These events took place in the month preceding surgery. She said she would not have the operation unless I was in the operating room during the surgery and in the recovery room after surgery. I made arrangements with the director of nursing and the operating room nursing supervisor and followed through with the nursing care in both units. She made the decision to go to Collingswood Nursing Center after hospitalization and I made several nursing home calls while she was there, especially on the day she wore her glasses for the first time.

Four months later, a cataract was removed from the right eye. In that instance, no house calls were needed prior to surgery or after the operation. I was in the operating room and recovery room as before, and the rest of the time the client exercised her self-care agency to the fullest and needed no professional nursing care. Her self-care assets included the ability to take full advantage of sources of professional help and an awareness of her nervous state. Her major deficit was her difficulty in coping with the fear of surgery the first time. The nursing care measure was assurance that I would be with her through all phases and that I could come if needed at any hour of the day or night. The outcome was that the client overcame her nervousness regarding the surgery, and that no additional nursing was needed at the time of the second operation.

Client example 12

When a mother and her 14-year-old son approached me for nursing care, I learned that the son had a diagnosis of leukemia and that the parents and an older son were addressing themselves to the task of coordinating multiple sets of information and many different medical people. They were anxious that the boy be helped to focus on what was strong in him, and that he use his assets in coping both with the knowledge that he would be under medical therapy for a long time and with the effects of medications, remissions and exacerbations. The whole family became my client collectively, and each member of the family became my client individually. Working with a family imposes unique demands in terms of meeting the needs of each and all, as these needs ebb and flow and storm within, in relation to the self and to the other members of the family. The self-care assets of the family as a whole included a strong love for and devotion to one another, bolstered by the assets of a high degree of intelligence and of a logic that permeated every deliberation in solving every crisis. Their humility in compliance, their distress when logic was being violated, their consideration of themselves as fallible judges even though they had facts in hand which ran counter to what was being medically effected for the boy—these served them well when they turned to me for assistance in helping them make a decision or in implementing a decision they had made.

I have chosen one of the hundreds of instances of nursing care given to this family to illustrate the concept of giving nursing care to a family as a unit. As their professional nurse, I went with them to the physician who was insisting that the boy leave the hospital because he had gone into remission for two-and-half days. The parents did not want to take the boy home, because the first doses of a new drug would then be given while he was out of the hospital. The parents wanted to see how he would react to the drug with medical care close by. They wanted the assurance of several blood tests a week—not just one—because of the rapidity with which their son's condition had changed. And they felt that they could take their son home only if the physicians could be more definitive in identifying the signs and symptoms that would herald at the earliest possible moment the need to return him to the hospital. A rather intense debate took place in the physician's office, since I remained firm on the conditions under which the parents felt they would take their son home. "We will not take John home until Miss Kinlein says it is all right for us to take him home," they said. This statement is historic in the perspective of the dissonance it reveals between the nursing care being given to the parents and the medical care being given to the son, and because of the parents' recognition that they had a need which required professional nursing care.

As a result of the meeting with the physician, the boy remained in the hospital for two-and-a-half more days and the other criteria set up by the parents were met prior to his discharge. The outcome of nursing care was that the boy and I achieved a unique relationship as he entered the final phase of the illness that culminated in his death. The nursing care of their son gave the parents much solace. The parents stated in 1975 and again in 1976 that the family would most probably have broken apart had it not received professional nursing care.

Client example 13

A 25-year-old woman sought my nursing care after she learned that her father had just been diagnosed as diabetic. She wanted information about the disease and about how she might be able to lessen her chances of developing it. I answered her questions, emphasized the importance of regular periodic tests of the blood and urine, analyzed her diet habits and suggested ways in which they might be improved in light of her concern.

On a subsequent visit she expressed concern about pressures associated with her job. She held a demanding professional position unusual for a woman her age, and felt that she was having difficulty coping with some of the problems of the job. I suggested that she keep a close record of the precise situations that produced anxiety, and I offered possible causes and suggested methods for coping with them. I also suggested exercises to reduce muscle tension and emphasized the importance of deep breathing and concentration on relaxation during anxious moments. During later appointments, with the anxiety-producing situations identified, we focused on measures for dealing with them. With nursing care the client was able to recognize that she lacked some of the trouble-shooting skills normally used in the business world. In subsequent appointments we worked on these skills—manner of speaking, tone of voice, gestures, behavior during meetings, methods of dealing with supervisors and subordinates in a way that would maintain respect and harmony. When a stress-producing situation was anticipated in advance, I would establish alternate methods and

concrete measures for handling it, so that the client could eliminate some of the unexpected in the situation and gain better
control of it. At each session she would recount situations indicating progress and a reduction in anxiety.

During one appointment she expressed con-
cern about pain she had been feeling for the past year in her
knee joints. Believing the problem might be cardiovascular, she
had visited a peripheral vascular specialist and had been told
that the problem was not cardiovascular. When she asked what
type of problem it might be, so that she could choose the appropriate specialist to consult, the physician told her it was "probably nothing." She discussed the situation with me, and nursing
care helped her to make the decision to see another doctor. She
asked me to question her about the symptoms, so that when she
saw the next physician she would be able to give him specific
descriptions of her symptoms. She visited an orthopedic surgeon
who, after hearing the symptoms, told her she was probably
paying too much attention to "little aches and pains." Because of
her knowledge of her symptoms, and because she was confident
of her judgments as a result of the nursing care she received, she
would not accept that response and told the physician, "I am
perfectly willing to accept that conclusion, but only when it is
based on actual tests." He responded that he would order some
blood work, "if it will make you feel any better." When she returned for the test results, the physician's attitude had changed.
The results indicated possible rheumatoid arthritis. He prescribed eight aspirin a day, even though she had indicated to
him in her medical history that aspirin irritated her stomach. He
changed the orders to Tylenol, told her to return in six weeks
and to call him "when there is any swelling." Realizing the potential seriousness of arthritis, the client indicated her dissatis-
faction with the medical regimen, and I supported her in her
judgment. She felt she should know more about how she might
decelerate the progress of the disease, rather than wait until
there was swelling to take action. She then consulted a rheumatologist who, she said, took the most complete medical history
she had ever encountered. He stressed the importance of good
health care habits, adequate rest, sensible eating practices and
reduced tension, and he taught her exercises to keep the joints

working and lubricated. So that the rheumatologist would have a more complete picture of her health state, she asked me to write him a letter for his file with my nursing judgments about her health. The physician prescribed sodium salicylate, which she was able to tolerate without any stomach upset. Her nursing care then focused on a sensible regimen of health maintenance in view of the disease. She returns to the rheumatologist every six months, and each time is able to report fewer pains. There has been no joint damage, and the physician has remarked that her ability to cope with stress and her self-confidence have both been greatly improved. She has progressed to the extent that she now needs no medication, and there has been no advancement of the disease.

The client's self-care assets included self-knowledge, the willingness to take steps to inform herself and then to verify that information with me, and the ability to integrate the scientific basis in changing her behavior patterns. The self-care deficits included the cyclic effect of a lack of confidence and the emergence of constantly challenging situations with new aspects—producing an improvement in self-confidence which was tenuous and needed to become solidified. The outcome has been the acquisition of self-confidence; an integrated view of herself—from the perspectives of woman, wife and professional person; and the manifestation to herself and others of a solid inner peace and strength that support her on a daily basis through the "rough spots." The client reports that she has never felt better in her personal and professional life and attributes this progress to the nursing care she received.

Client example 14

A woman in her forties came to see me because someone had urged her to seek my nursing care. She was on various illegal drugs and on alcohol, and had been thinking of suicide. She said she doubted I could help her, and I said I did not know yet whether or not I could.

She spoke tersely in sentences of three or four words, her lips held tightly and her mouth barely moving. It was very difficult to understand her. Her eyes had a look combining fear, defiance and hate, giving the overall impression of a steely-eyed individual who would challenge anyone who jarred her. At times, a pleading look would appear and disappear. As I listened, her eyes were penetrating, as if in search of evidence to determine if she could place her trust in me.

Her most obvious self-care asset was the mustering of courage to try to get help—again—despite the burden of layers of past failures weighting her will to the point of despair and annihilation. Because of her staccato manner of speaking, the obvious difficulty she had in expressing herself and her wary attitude, I decided to prescribe a nursing measure to help her describe more easily her state of mind and body. At the end of the appointment I prescribed a nursing care measure consisting of exercises of the facial muscles, especially the orbicularis oris. Her manner of blocking visible signs of reaction on her part left me in doubt about the efficacy of my efforts, and I had no way of knowing her reaction to the nursing care prescription. Finally she said, "You think that would help, huh? . . . You know I am more relaxed with you than I am at home or elsewhere." I had previously mentioned that she ground her teeth together when she was especially tense. "You should hear me grind my teeth at home," she now said.

It was impossible for me to identify other self-care assets and deficits during this first appointment, because I had to move so slowly with her, carefully guiding her to open up. She blocked too much to enable me to make any other judgments about self-care assets and deficits, even though the appointment was two hours long.

In this case, the hazard of leaping to conclusions about the cause of her problems was an extreme one. I had the sensation of being in an intellectual environment that had no gravity, and I had no way of knowing how effective I had been. This case surely would challenge an experienced person and so would be classified as a complex nursing situation with respect to the curriculum level.

Would she ask for another appointment? I had no way of knowing. A month later, she did call to make another appointment.

During our second visit, she said she had

been very upset during the initial appointment, and was even more upset now. She related that she had just been fired because she had come to work in a drunken state. She recalled the details of the evening leading up to the firing, and related things in a much more relaxed manner than she had the first time. In the absence of any evidence to the contrary, I could only assume that she had developed trust in me.

This time, she demonstrated self-care assets that included the ability to listen and to try to analyze without a wall of protective defiance blocking both my words and her own. She reported that she had also stopped using drugs for several months. However, as she talked I sensed that she was somewhat obsessed with the notion that she could not stay off the drugs.

The appointment progressed quite satisfactorily and lasted two-and-a-half hours. The analysis evolved into an acceptance by her that a physiological aberration existed which needed exploration. Several years before she had had a glucose tolerance test that indicated the presence of hypoglycemia. She had put herself on a diet, but refused to seek medical care. During this appointment she said firmly that she would not pursue medical treatment. I accepted that, and drew for her, as the appointment progressed, a diagram illustrating her position (page 168).

The situation, reduced to its narrowest terms, was a matter of her choosing life or death. I explained that if she chose life, it would involve remaining off drugs, exploring the metabolic aberration, and obtaining another job, and that I would help her through these by establishing self-care measures with her and by providing support. However, if she chose death, then there were other arrangements that she would have to make. "You have the free will to decide," I said to her. She was quiet for several minutes. "Suppose I can't find out what's wrong with me?" she asked. When I continued to explain the possible benefits of seeking medical care, she narrowed her eyes and said to me, "How can you encourage me to see a doctor so I will feel better, when I say it is no use to go, and on the other hand, a while back you said you would help me if I chose to die?" I replied, "Because you made the decision to seek life, not to seek

I have used this approach with clients who introduce the notion of suicide in their alternative plans. I tell them I will help them make the decision in regard to choosing between life and death. I explore with them the following questions:

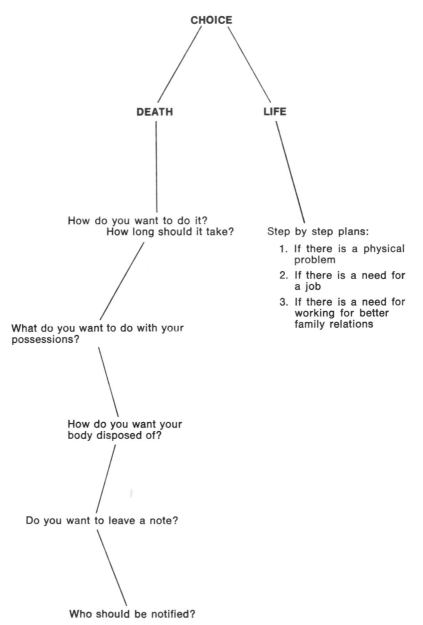

CHOICE

DEATH

How do you want to do it?
How long should it take?

What do you want to do with your possessions?

How do you want your body disposed of?

Do you want to leave a note?

Who should be notified?

LIFE

Step by step plans:

1. If there is a physical problem

2. If there is a need for a job

3. If there is a need for working for better family relations

death." And I turned back the pages of my notebook to the section in which she had worked through the decision. There was a moment of silence while this sank in, and then a slow smile spread across her face. She changed her position in the chair—she stretched out somewhat. I followed up with, "I will support you in the decisions you make." She added, "You realize that if you make me accountable for what I do, then the burden is on me. I will be exercising my self-care agency in what I do."

The nursing care measures at this point were for her to record her thinking process in considering her reasons for a block against medical care, to continue with the diet that she said made her feel better, and to engage in exercise and sports activities to counteract the fatigue she reported. The major self-care deficit that has to be worked with is her inability to take steps in light of her decision to seek life.

At the end of the second appointment she said she was frightened when people were near to her and might know about her situation. I encouraged her to voice such feelings because it would help her to see her own self-image and to deal with the embarrassment she feels. This is a possible starting point for her at the next appointment.

Client example 15

Another client, a woman in her thirties, came to me because she had discovered a lump in her breast and was faced with the prospect of a mastectomy. I helped her through the decision-making process, during which she chose to have a biopsy operation only, followed by a modified mastectomy, with removal of some lymph nodes. The nursing care measures that I have taken have consisted primarily of giving her factual information and encouraging her to pursue all her concerns even in the face of many hurdles. She has contacted many individuals in the medical field as she pursued to a conclusion the details she could not at first understand. Her greatest concern was the maintenance of a self-image that would not be misunderstood by the many individuals she contacted in her search for answers. Above all, she said, she did not want to be seen as a "hysterical woman."

The postoperative period was relatively smooth for her because she had proceeded in a very deliberate, circumspect manner in regard to getting additional medical opinions about the surgical therapy for breast cancer and about follow-up care. But despite all of this preparation, she continued to need help as she approached the time for viewing the incision, wearing a prosthesis and resuming everyday activities. For a time, there was stress in the family, and she needed help in attaining a state of serenity in her relationship with her husband and children. I have been giving her nursing care for a period of six months, and she anticipates that she will continue to need nursing care. At her request, I forwarded to her physician the following résumé of her nursing progress:

> An appraisal of her needs in all phases of her care disclosed the pattern of:
> 1. Auditory reception of the words *cancer, surgery, mastectomy, recovery*
> 2. Comprehension of the fact that the words were about her, and not the many other patients she has cared for
> 3. A somewhat stoic, logical reaction following the comprehension about herself, followed by
> 4. An appropriate indulgence in the soothing feeling of introspective analysis of her feelings as she reviewed the past events
>
> Her self-care assets throughout were the maintenance of wariness about feeling self-pity; searching out facts and resources so she could make better decisions; cautiously testing her readiness to engage in certain activities; admission of the strain on the family as well as on herself; and asking for help in minimizing that strain and restoring an atmosphere of harmony and understanding in the house. A need (of my client) is to have all the pieces of a complex picture accounted for and put in place before she can move through the difficult period of adjustment to a more placid state of being.

The client now is more calm in her manner, and reports that she thinks first before responding and doesn't "fly off the handle as much." She is now able to look at her incision and to talk about the mastectomy. She says that she can see the progress she is making every day in coping with this situation.

Client example 16

When the mother of an eight-year-old boy called for an appointment with me, she indicated that her son had asthma and that she wanted me to see him. The physicians had said the cause of the asthma was emotional, that no treatment was necessary, and that he would outgrow it eventually. The mother said, "What I want to know is: what do I do while he is outgrowing it?"

When she came for the appointment she brought both of her sons, and discussed freely in their presence her marital state (she had recently been divorced), the rivalry between the two boys, and her job. I gathered what she told me into a picture of the family group and indicated that at first the focus would be on the younger son, since he seemed to be most in need of the family's support at that time. I told all three of them that anything that took place or was said during the appointments with the young son would be held in strictest confidence, and that I would first ask the son's permission before I talked about it to his mother or anyone else. The boy listened intently, and on the next appointment he came alone. He brought his stethoscope and I listened to his chest through his stethoscope and then through mine. I graphed the nature of his breathing and started him on a series of exercises to relax his muscles of respiration. Subsequently, I tested his breathing responses to physical activity by playing ball with him. He talked about his different feelings when he was "sort of" sick and when he was very sick, and he kept an account of how he felt for a three-week period by putting different colored stars on a sheet of paper. He was making progress in his ability to relax his muscles when he was having difficulty breathing.

His self-care assets were that he was able to integrate what I was suggesting into his daily activities and that he could also make distinctions about what I was talking about concerning his care. He always took seriously everything I said.

One day, his mother brought him for another appointment. I heard her voice as she approached the door. It was extremely agitated in tone, and she talked very rapidly. When they came into my office, it was obvious that the mother was upset. Her eyes were flashing, her nostrils flaring, her movements very brusque. "Oh, that man!" she said. "I hate him. . . . I hate him. . . . I just came from seeing ————'s father. . . . He is impossible . . . and all the trouble I've had at the house . . . that man is just . . . I could kill him. . . . I really could kill him. . . . I'm not kidding, Miss Kinlein, I could kill him." As his mother talked, the child's breathing, which was labored when he came in, grew worse. There were the inspiratory wheeze and the look of panic that accompany the event of status asthmaticus. I said softly to the mother, "You are upset. Would you like me to give you a back rub? I think it would make you feel more comfortable, more relaxed." "Oh, that sounds wonderful. But this is ————'s appointment. I don't want to take his time." I smiled at the child and said, "I don't think he would mind if I gave you a back rub to soothe you." The child nodded his approval. I took his mother into my examining room and gave her a back rub— the most therapeutic back rub I have given in my nursing career. As I proceeded with the back rub, the mother's voice became softer. She became somewhat relaxed, and as the noise level lowered in the office, I listened for her son's breathing. It, too, was calmer, and the wheezing sounds had subsided. "I feel so much better," his mother said. "I'll leave you with ———— so he can have his appointment."

The child and I continued with the nursing measures that had been started. He talked to me and we worked on his exercises. His mother later said he was doing better in school and seemed more relaxed. He said, "When I get excited I do as you told me, and it helps."

The son improved, but the family moved and I have not seen them since the initial nursing care in 1972–73. I must point out, however, that during that time, in the early years of my practice, I was still somewhat hemmed in by the medical model and concentrated on the physiological aspects of this client case. I did not feel free enough to attempt to give nursing care with respect to the relationship between the mother and the son, an important factor, I knew, in the child's problems. Now, as my nursing care has developed, I would propose nursing measures for the mother as well—measures designed to help her understand her role in the situation and to take steps to make improvements aimed at producing a healthier family environment for her sons and for herself.

Client example 17

A man in his late sixties asked for my nursing care when he became concerned about itching and dryness in his right ear. By examining his ear I determined that the condition did not signal a need for medical care. He told me he had been using a patent medicine that was giving him very little relief, and we then discussed other possibilities, including the use of baby oil. When the itching was prolonged and intense, there was some minor scabbing in the canal. I suggested cleansing the area with a mild antiseptic and, after careful drying of the area, applying baby oil. The condition would get better, then come back. He tried other remedies, one of which his son had used for the same dryness and itching of the ear. The client decided not to see a physician and said confidently that the condition would clear up. Eventually, the condition did clear up and the problem has not recurred.

Recently the client's wife made an appointment for a partial physical examination. She said she was feeling well and wanted to know more about her health state. Her husband and two-and-a-half-year-old granddaughter accompanied her to the appointment. The husband, too, will be returning for a physical examination for the same reason.

The client's self-care assets were that he had knowledge of his physical state and was able to take action in light of this knowledge of himself and of his ear condition. When he called me to discuss a possible new remedy he was considering trying, he had thought out specific questions and was able to incorporate the answers into his decision-making process in a sensible way. One of his self-care deficits was a small degree of uncertainty about the nature of the ear condition and his approach in trying to remedy it. Nursing care measures included giving him support in his decisions regarding his approach to the condition when they were based on fact and sound judgment, and watching for any change in the appearance of the dryness and itching. The outcome was that the client was able to pursue this particular problem with confidence and without anxiety to a successful end, and that his general health state is being improved through his desire to seek nursing care and his ability to make good use of the information he receives.

Client example 18

The granddaughter of a 94-year-old client asked me to make a house call to see her grandmother. She wanted to see if something could be done to strengthen her grandmother's leg muscles. The grandmother had walked a great deal until several months ago, when she seemed to lose strength in her legs and as a result stopped her exercise of walking. The granddaughter asked me to initiate any measures that would help her grandmother retain the health she had.

After examining the grandmother I designed a system of nursing care for her. Practical nurses care for her on a 24-hour basis and follow through with the nursing measures I prescribe in the design of the nursing system for my client. In this instance, the clients to whom I give nursing care are the granddaughter and her mother, and nursing care at a technical level is given to the grandmother. I demonstrate to the practical nurses the kind of exercises she should receive; I answer their questions and discuss aspects of the grandmother's care with them. The nursing measures that I established in light of the results of the physical examination were:

—Passive exercises to restore a degree of muscle tone to her legs

—Small, frequent feedings to maintain good physical state through sound nutritional habits

—Increased ingestion or iron to improve her blood picture, which showed a low red blood cell count, low hemoglobin, and low hematocrit

—Exercises of the lungs to increase their capacity and decrease the chances of fluid accumulation

—Instituting no measures during the brief episodes of absence of heartbeat. Her heart has so far picked up its beat after a temporary halt; there is no measure that can be taken in this instance that will reinstitute the beat.

In assisting the granddaughter and her mother in the care of the elderly woman, I built upon the self-care assets of: love for the woman, which has enabled them to seek measures and take action to insure her comfort; and their knowledge about the physiology and nutritional needs of an elderly person. Nursing care measures for them included the assurance that their relative was getting excellent care, through explanations of the nature of that care; and the assurance that I was always within reach to answer any questions or to come to see any member of the family to give nursing care.

Client example 19

A client came to me because she wanted to become pregnant. She had been to many specialists and said she had tried "everything" that was recommended to her by them. In addition, she had read widely on the subject of infertility.

When she came to me she was nervous and concerned that her state of mind might become obsessive, and also that her husband might have to consider the possibility that he was sterile. She was trying to spare him the trauma of that consideration as long as possible.

Her self-care assets were her relentless search for information that might help in her effort to become pregnant and her total willingness to keep trying, even measures that had been tried before. Nursing care measures included the suggestion that she position her hips on a pillow during sexual intercourse to supply gravitational assistance to the movement of the sperm; that she and her husband prolong postcoital closeness and affection, with a view to the attainment of a second orgasm, if possible; that she and her husband take special care to delay his climax until she was very much ready; that she talk over with her husband the methods of fondling that she finds very satisfying, since it is possible that she was trying so hard to become pregnant from a scientific perspective that she was unconsciously withholding the most essential ingredient of the expression of love between her and her husband—total abandonment; which might contribute the yet-to-be-identified element that total physical and psychological relaxation supplies in the process of conception.

We talked about how her priority of motherhood might demand the sacrifice of her job, which she enjoyed very much. In light of her expressed belief in God, we also discussed the possibility that God, in His wisdom and love, might not want to give her a child, and that this might be what she was being asked to accept. She said that this viewpoint had not been proposed to her before and that she began to feel better about everything. The following year the client became pregnant and subsequently delivered a normal, healthy baby.

Client example 20

Some of the clients who have come to me because of their concern about their blood pressure reading can be discussed from the point of view of classification of their expression of need, the self-care assets at work and the nursing care measures instituted in light of them. This particular group of clients consists of men from the ages of 28 to 75.

Client A

"I wonder what my blood pressure is," one man said. "I think it must be normal." The client continued to talk about his general health state, declaring he was not really worried about his blood pressure, but felt he should know that parameter of his state of health, just as he knew other points about himself. He knew, for example, that he ate well, slept well and enjoyed his work and life in general. We discussed the details of his self-care practices, and the self-care assets that emerged were his accurate knowledge of nutrition and the integration of good health measures into his pattern of living. After taking his blood pressure and discussing the results with him, the nursing care measures consisted of an endorsement of his

current judgments and actions and a recommendation to learn
to a greater degree the salutary effect of conscious control of
blood pressure in stress-producing situations. The ways to control blood pressure were discussed fully with him. At subsequent
appointments, he said he felt much better about the whole
physiological phenomenon of blood pressure and also everyday
living.

Client B

Another client came to me saying, "I don't
really think this medicine helps my blood pressure that much.
Sometimes I just stop taking it. And then I start again." The
drug was Lasix. In the ensuing discussion the client noted that
sometimes he got weak and shaky, and that scared him. I
pointed out to him the effects of loss of potassium and named
some foods high in potassium that he might consider eating. His
daily practices included ingestion of large amounts of alcohol
and salty foods, and he indicated that he was aware of the
effects of such a diet. His outlook on life was negative, and he
felt despondent.

His greatest self-care asset was his basic hu-
mility about himself, which enabled him to see the contradictory
practices he engaged in. Nursing care measures included exploration of his health goals and his outlook on life. After seven
or eight months, which included six appointments, his outlook
had improved, he had lost weight, and although his blood pressure had come down only several points, he said he was feeling
better. This client continues to make appointments for nursing
care.

Client C

A client in his seventies was taking care of
his elderly wife, who was a semi-invalid. He had had difficulty
obtaining adequate medical care for both of them, and this was
a concern to him. His wife's need for nursing care placed a
physical strain on him when he tried to give her the care, and a
financial strain when he had to pay for nurses. This man was a
retired engineer and a person who was very sensitive and self-
disciplined. His apprehension about his wife's comfort, the gen-

eral lack of interest displayed toward him when he tried to meet his needs in a logical fashion (for example, unnecessarily long waiting periods for medication when he had planned to accomplish other errands early on a hot summer day), and the callousness of people he had to deal with all made him very upset. Then he would worry about getting a stroke and ask, "What would happen to my wife?" This worry about getting a stroke would manifest itself when I entered the house. The husband would say, "Before you start with my wife, will you take my blood pressure? I'm sure it's very high." I would then talk with him and help him to relax. In this instance, the danger was bidirectional. If I took his blood pressure when it was high, and told him the results (which is an integral aspect of my nursing care), he would then worry more. On the other hand, waiting too long to take it could produce a state of anxiety because of his urgent need to know it right away. As the husband and I talked, I watched for signals that would indicate the best time to take the blood pressure—after he was more relaxed, but before he had become too anxious—and then take his blood pressure reading.

His self-care assets included his planning for rest periods for himself and his attempt to accept philosophically that which he could not change. Nursing care measures included rendering physical care to his wife initially, and then getting a practical nurse for her on a continuing basis; helping him when he felt the need to cry; and giving him support in the decisions he had to make about his wife and himself. Eventually, his wife was placed in a nursing home and died two years later.

Client D

This client had gone to a medical center in response to publicity announcing that participants were being sought for a study of coronary risk factors. The criteria for admission to the study included a high blood pressure reading and a high cholesterol level. The client was certain that he would be accepted for the study.

There was a mixture of jubilation and disappointment in his voice when he told me he had not been accepted for the study. I pointed out that it was a medical study about disease-prone individuals, testing the knowledge that the physicians had at the present time about coronary heart disease. After talking about it, he said he recognized the subtle irony in the whole situation of not being *sick* enough to participate in a study that *might* cast light on prevention of disease. He said that studying healthier individuals might yield more fruitful data, less likely to be obscured by concurrent pathology caused by the highly elevated blood pressure and cholesterol level.

The client's self-care assets were an increase in understanding of the part that physiological parameters play in the approach to care from a medical perspective and the approach to care from the nursing perspective—which emphasizes what is healthy in an individual as a point of departure, as opposed to what is less healthy. Through nursing care measures, which included the application of logic to the viewpoints of the two different professions, the client moved from a rather fatalistic outlook about the inevitability of a diseased condition, to a more positive approach, which included health care measures such as reducing his weight, cutting back on his alcohol intake and developing a happier attitude about his work situation.

At this point I must offer a comment about the male clients I have seen in my practice. It is hazardous to draw any conclusions now, but a hypothesis seems to be emerging in regard to the psychology of a man and his care of himself on a daily basis. In my practice it has been my experience that men have needed assistance in acquiring a degree of comfort in talking about a state of physical and mental health *in themselves*. I have noted a tendency on the part of my male clients to externalize measures and to minimize their own personalities in regard to those measures. If a degree of comfort is not achieved through nursing care during the client session, then the effectiveness of nursing measures implemented is proportionately impaired.

Client example 21

One of my clients, a woman in her early forties, came for nursing care because she said she wanted to feel more energetic. Her physician had said there was nothing wrong with her and had told her to stop doing so much, to "cut out a few activities."

In examining her daily activities with her, several points emerged. Her diet was composed of too many carbohydrates and starches and not enough protein and vitamins. In addition, she had developed a pattern of putting off household chores until they reached overwhelming proportions. Her self-care assets included an awareness of the need to take action if change was to occur in her health state.

At her request, I conducted a physical examination and drew blood for a study of her health profile. She was slightly anemic, so she began to take iron pills. I suggested that she select a special interest she had and she responded that she was very much interested in antique furniture. A nursing measure I prescribed was to go to the library at least once a week and read about antique furniture. Another nursing measure was to include in her diet more foods with a higher protein and vitamin content.

When she returned for subsequent appointments, she had lost some weight, her color was better, and she seemed more animated than before. She remarked that she felt better, and said it was "kind of funny. The doctor told me to eliminate one or two of my activities and you suggested adding one more to my list—to do more than I was doing. And I feel better. Of course, helping me with getting organized is good, and my diet does make me feel more energetic. I'm glad to lose the weight, too."

One day this client made an appointment because her beautician had said she found fleas in her hair. I examined her hair and told her it was pediculosis. I gave her the name of an over-the-counter remedy specific for this condition and told her about fumigating her furniture. Because of her interest in animals, she thought the problem must have been fleas. Also, she could not understand where she might have picked up the lice. She took some of the specimens to the Department of Agriculture and the report came back with the identification of pediculosis. She was embarrassed at having this condition and still puzzled about how she got it. She had mentioned on a previous occasion that she enjoyed yard sales, and I suggested that fabrics, such as those used in the sweaters and coats she purchased, could have harbored the lice. I also mentioned that cloth seats in public places could harbor lice.

Client example 22

Some clients have come to me because they were experiencing difficulties in relation to another person—specifically, their housemate or spouse. In all instances, the reason for coming was either to prevent marital problems, to deal with incipient ones, or to verify the status of their feelings concerning the need for separation. In each case, one member of the couple contacted me first, and subsequently both persons came, although each one had some appointments with me alone. Often, one would go window-shopping at a nearby shopping center while the other was with me, and then they would meet together at the end of the session. From the first contact, I approached the need as expressed by the individual in the framework of self-care practices, and it is astonishing how effective this approach is in the face of what one would call a marital problem.

Client A

In fact, an example of a nursing emergency could be given in the instance of the couple described on page 145 in Client Example 3. The young woman made an appointment to discuss the impending split with the father of her child. She asked for the appointment right away because she said she needed to talk about the situation, and needed help in following through with her plans. When she came to the office, however, she began to give me reasons for delaying the split. The reasons centered around the fact that she still loved the man, that she wanted her baby to know his father, and that she would marry him if he would stop being "inconsiderate" to her and getting angry with the baby when he cried. She said that she told him, "We are adults and ———— is a baby, completely egocentric, and it is up to us to teach him understanding and kindness and love. . . . Miss Kinlein, where can the cycle be ended and the start made? Why can't people see it? It is so obvious that you can't be a child forever, that you have to grow up and take responsibility. This baby is ours and we have to be responsible for him. Why can't he see that? I don't ask for anything in our togetherness except thoughtfulness and consideration . . . to be around to help me, not to go off to parties or off with his friends . . . there is more to life than that. Why can't people see that babies can't be hurt or the whole cycle will start all over again the next generation?" I replied, "You are asking the questions that confused Confucius."

This appointment is an example of a nursing emergency in that the client had to talk about the fact that instead of working through the intended separation, she was now working through the possibility of a legitimate married state. At the end of the hour-long appointment, I had another client appointment by telephone. The need of the first client was such that more time was needed, so I asked if she wanted to wait until after my next appointment to resume the nursing session. She eagerly agreed and so took care of the baby and wrote letters until one-and-a-half hours later, when we could resume the appointment. The baby who is my client (his mother acting as substitute agent), was in the office all the time, and I had an opportunity to assess his mother's care of him and to observe his excellent physiological and psychological state. When I gave them a ride home, because the child's father was out looking for a job, the client showed me some plants she was growing, including one that was for me. As I left, the father came home and we exchanged pleasantries. My client has asked him to come to me for assistance through this difficult period, but he has refused. Before her pregnancy, he had come with her for an appointment and had commented afterward how much I had helped them both.

The self-care assets the client has are her absolute ability to see and analyze a situation clearly, her psychological strength, and her lack of self-pity. This last trait, however, is almost simultaneously a self-care deficit. She guards so strongly against self-pity that she put herself last, in spite of the numerous physical complications she has experienced. This sometimes gives her an unrealistic view of the facts, and prevents her from being able to see when her own health is at stake. She is willing to put her own health in jeopardy unnecessarily.

Some nursing care measures include trying to find ways to help her mate understand for himself the need to be considerate and responsible, instead of telling him what he should or should not be doing; and relying on her own strength in taking the initiative to improve the relationship. She has decided to work with him in this regard. "I would marry him then; I would be at peace," she said. "But I won't let him marry me because of pressure from our parents." This situation will require ongoing nursing care.

Client B

A husband and wife came to see me because they wanted their marriage to remain intact. There were misunderstandings about each other's needs, they felt, and they wanted to iron them out so that the marriage could be happier. The fact that the wife was on the pill entered the picture, as is so often the case with couples who have sought my nursing care in regard to marital problems. Generally, more concern is expressed about the loss of libido, than is expressed about the possibility of clots, strokes, etc. One of the most enlightening points of discussion for the couple is to see the bitter irony in the fact that the pill was intended to "free" the woman from the burden of unwanted pregnancy, and hence to create a more satisfying physical effect during intercourse—thereby improving the marital relationship because the woman enjoys the intimate affection much more. Now, many couples have had to come to grips with the fact that in many instances, the pill has created a distaste for intimacy because the wife often cannot even muster a desire, no matter how much she tries. Many have said to me, "I used to be able to talk myself into it, but now I can't even do that." The self-care assets and deficits vary in each instance, of course, but in all the cases, the value of working through one's own self-care in light of values and goals has brought about change in one partner and then invariably in the other.

In giving nursing care to the wife, the self-care assets that emerged were her view of herself as an individual, her sincere effort to behave in consonance with the goal of a happy marriage, and her ability to accept the truth about herself. The self-care deficits were that she wanted to be married and to have a happy marriage, but also had the attitude that "I want to do what I want to do." She also lacked an appreciation of her husband's viewpoint and of the give-and-take nature of marriage itself.

Nursing care measures were to relax in hot baths—together or alone—and to engage in exercises, in an effort to improve their sexual relations. A method was also suggested for dealing with situations that aroused anger in one or the other of them. The disturbed partner was to say, "I am bothered about something and I want to talk about it." If the other replied, "Not now," then the wife or husband would ask, "Then when can we discuss it?" And the other person would have to make a commitment to have the discussion at a certain time. Also, when they became very angry with one another, it was suggested that they look into each other's eyes, smile and touch each other—not necessarily in an embrace, but simply to make contact—as in touching the shoulder or elbow. The encounter usually provided time for cooling off, the eye contact symbolized the desire on the part of each to communicate with the other, and the touching served as a reminder of the affection that existed, in spite of the current bone of contention between them. This approach worked with this couple during one nursing session, when they became angry. The wife reached over and touched the husband, who then put his arm around her. I said quietly, "Let yourself fall into his arms. I'll go in the other room." I left them alone for a few minutes. They remained in each other's arms and tears were in their eyes. When I returned, they were still in each other's arms, not crying, but simply relaxing.

Other nursing care measures were to develop criteria regarding the subject matter of arguments—to ask themselves, "Is this a spark, or a flame? Is this important enough to pursue?" This would enable each to arrive at a point where it was possible to say, "I think I can let this go by," and to focus on what was really important. It was also suggested that each partner concentrate on developing a sense of humor and the ability to laugh at himself or herself more, to lessen concern with vulnerability as well as defensiveness.

In every instance there has been an improvement in the relationship. The couple would call me and say something like this: "Things have been going just beautifully since our last appointment. We want to make another appointment for two weeks from now."

Who can say when nursing care has been effective in marital situations? The nature of marriage is such that daily appraisal of its state must be carried out by both partners.

Client C

I have mentioned previously that the time element is crucial in giving nursing care. The importance of this factor emerged in the nursing care given during a session with one married couple. Had I terminated the session at the end of the appointed time, their problems of mutual misunderstanding would have been compounded.

I have been caring for the wife since November, 1975 and the husband and wife together since January, 1976. A two-hour appointment had been scheduled and was proceeding quite well. Although progress was apparent and they both realized it, evidence emerged that the wife was not fully satisfied that her husband understood how she felt about the main issue of planning in light of the changes that had taken place in their lives. To the husband, the points that had been made were very clear, and he understood the need for his wife to know what point his thinking had reached in regard to his work and school.

But something else lingered that was fundamental to so many of their problems in the past. My dilemma was this: If I pursued the concerns of the wife, I was going to have to take an approach that would open up another lengthy analysis, and I sensed that the husband had felt that the session was concluded after two hours and ten minutes has passed. In addition, I knew I would have to point out the wife's self-care deficits in regard to planning, and I had to assess the effect this would have on the gains that had been made in the understanding between the two of them concerning *her valid points about him*. My nursing approach was this: I made some changes in my physical position, I leaned forward as I talked, I would half close my book and then open it again to write or to draw a point for clarification. Thus, the viewpoints of both husband and wife were being served simultaneously in my judgment. As the wife continued to talk, one of her very persistent traits was isolated and discussed, and the influence of this trait on the past relationship came to light. The husband, his interest reawakened, participated in the exchange by lovingly disclosing some details, examples and explanations of the points I was making to her. When the husband looked at his watch at 11:05 P.M., he remarked: "An hour ago, I thought we had expended the profit of this session and had gone ten minutes past the profit point. Now, I think we made extraordinary progress in the last 40 minutes or less! Isn't it interesting how it works?"

The wife eventually acknowledged the logic of her self-care deficit, which I had put forth with extreme care. She then worked with plans that were based on the recognized fact of her persistent deficit. At the door, the husband said, "I don't know when would be a good time for the next appointment, but we'll make one." They went down the hall, hand in hand.

I try to leave cushions of time in making appointments when I think that the need of my clients will unfold slowly. Giving effective nursing care demands extended periods of time.

Client D

A woman asked for nursing care in regard to her imminent separation from her husband, whom she still loved very much. In the initial appointments, the client cried a lot and had a difficult time working through her anger at her husband and the hostility she felt because of the way life had treated her. She suggested to her husband that he come for nursing care, and he agreed. The joint appointment was kept and afterward the husband agreed to make subsequent appointments.

The wife's self-care assets included her ability to face the fact that she would have to adjust to her husband's infidelity and inability to reverse the trend he was taking

—which was leading to the dissolution of their marriage—even though he tried and was upset that he could not take the steps leading to a reconciliation. Her major self-care deficit was her poor self-image, which became worse as the marriage deteriorated. One of the nursing care measures was to support my client in the notion that she could change her self-image. She feared that she would take the route of promiscuity. One of my statements that she indicated helped her was: "People change; *you* can change." She told me she kept repeating that to herself and was able to take steps that would lead ultimately to her acquiring a master's degree and a good position. The client has now regained some of the weight she had lost, no longer has dark circles under her eyes and presents a far more serene picture than she did before. In addition, she does not cry as much as she did before. She proceeded with the divorce, although her husband said he wanted to come back to her. She said, "Miss Kinlein, it would be the same thing all over again in another year or two. That's the way it always has been. It's time he realized he has to change, to grow up. This time it's different."

I have helped individuals with respect to relationships with persons of the opposite sex, regardless of the client's set of values, philosophy or view of spiritual matters. For example, I have given care to a person who is an atheist, but who found stability and strength in his view of me as a deeply spiritual and religious person. This particular client had been to therapists, psychiatrists and counselors. He maintained that he had been helped only very slightly by the others, but found that I was able to help him most. He suggested that two other persons come to see me as a result of his progress with my nursing care.

When an issue is judgmental, I do not impose my values on the client. I give views based on professional knowledge. This client told me, "Until you told me you were a Roman Catholic, I didn't know it." I believe it comes through therapeutically that I have certain values; I have a stability in those values and a message of self-discipline comes through. This trait in the professional nurse gives people a standard of comparison, a reference point they can use in assessing and understanding their own needs.

The essence of nursing care with respect to personal relationships—and to all needs, actually—lies in how the professional nurse says what she says and when she says it. It lies in knowing when the clients are ready to hear the words, when they are able to integrate them, and when they are ready to translate their understanding into action. The difficulty lies in meeting the needs of two persons simultaneously. Yet I have witnessed self-care awareness unfold before my eyes, as the crucial moment for something to be processed within the person's being is reached. Self-care assets and deficits are clearly revealed in a session in which two individuals are attempting to express their individual needs and their needs as a couple.

Client example 23

Several clients I have seen in my practice have had their living patterns changed because of "back pain." If there is one single pathological state that can be prevented in almost all instances, it is the back pain that is caused either by trauma produced in the muscles of the lumbar or sacral region, or by the intermittently ruptured or permanently ruptured nucleus pulposus of the intervertebral disc. The clients in my practice have been both male and female and all have been past the age of 30. The significance of the fact that this condition is preventable should make the nursing profession realize that the lack of nursing care prior to the appearance of back pain may account for the percentage of incidence every year in the United States.

If, for example, individuals had access to a professional nurse's services for the purpose of learning body mechanics and posture (as a control in the activities of lifting and pulling, pushing and moving, getting in and out of a chair, picking up a thread from the floor, reinforcing the body against the explosive force that accompanies a sneeze or a cough, the incidence of "back pain" as a medical condition requiring hours of treatment would diminish dramatically. In addition, the ways of treating minor discomfort and pain in muscles that have not been used, and that are then put to use in either sports or household activities, can be implemented by the lay person, resulting in a marked reduction in the number of days spent in discomfort and the time spent away from work. This muscular and neural condition is certainly a prime example of a truism that is generally accepted but rarely observed in practice: Knowledge is the prevention, knowledge is the treatment, knowledge will set you free of pain in this situuation.

Client A

A 66-year-old man had been treated by a succession of specialists in the medical field. There had been no lasting cure of his ailment. He showed me the diagnosis of ruptured intervertebral disc, which, he said, "the doctor wrote down because he did not know how else to assure that I could collect Medicare for all the expenses." As I proceeded in my nursing care of the client, he asked me if he could relieve his pain in any way, since he did not like to take medication all the time, which was all the doctors could offer him for relief. I listened to his description of his pain, of the temporary relief he had received from acupuncture, from a chiropractor, and from the use of his own good judgment. I set up a series of exercises that I usually prescribe for clients with the same need, and I demonstrated these exercises to him. Of course, each client has different needs in terms of ability to perform the exercises, the time needed to incorporate them into his daily schedule, the accuracy with which the exercises are carried out, and the assistance needed to provide enough motivation to remain faithful to the observance of the basic actions to the point that they will be unconsciously applied in the measures of everyday living. It is as difficult to change a habit of posture as it is to change a habit of smoking, of drinking, or of biting one's nails.

The positional aids helped my client so much that in a few weeks he called to tell me how much better he felt. A period of eleven months had elapsed and there has been no recurrence of the pain that plagued him when he was in bed, that bothered him while getting up and moving about during the day, and that made him cry in misery. A description of the general nature of the exercises follows.

Nursing care measures

I. EXERCISES—3x a day for 10 minutes:
1. Standing: Retract abdominal muscles and contract gluteal muscles (buttocks) and hold to the count of 5. Relax completely for count of 5. Repeat each step for the 10 minutes.
2. Breathe normally throughout the exercises. Be sure to coordinate breathing and exercises. The muscles need the oxygen.

II. EXERCISES—3x a day for 20 minutes:
1. Lie on floor with small pillow under your head, feet in chair; use rolled magazines and heating pad. Turn heating pad on "low" and place between the rolled magazines and back.
2. *It is important to relax* during this exercise. Heat to the muscles will further increase relaxation and ease the contraction that causes more pressure on the nerve.

III. IN GENERAL—Keep back straight while turning over after the exercises. Use your tightened buttock muscles and tightened abdominal muscles to keep your back in the straight position as you roll over. Use arm muscles and leg muscles to take the strain.

Remember:
1. Move slowly and deliberately at all times.
2. Use your own judgment; there is evidence that you make sound judgments about your back.
3. If you consult a physician, ask for his reasons for the medical care.

Client B

A woman in her forties came to me because she had not slept for two weeks as a result of intense pain when she lay in bed. In the office, she explained to me the nature of the pain, the exact point at which the pain had appeared, and the other areas to which it had moved—across her back and down her leg. This client had come to see me previously for other reasons, and as she had done in the past, she had written down all the details of the appearance of the condition. She had consulted a physician and he had said the back pain was from tension. He had prescribed Valium and an analgesic. She had described the episodes of pain as being similar to "spasms." I listened to her, and I asked her to tell me, if she could, exactly when the pain appeared the first time. She replied, "Oh, yes, I can tell you exactly when." She stood up with difficulty and demonstrated how she had pushed back a line of clothes on a rack in a department store to get at a box a customer had come pick up. As I watched her, I observed her body, bent from the waist, out of alignment, and twisted as she pantomimed moving the clothes on the rack. As her body remained twisted when she bent to pick up the box for the customer in her demonstration, I envisioned the strain on her back and I could almost hear the nucleus pulposus slip out. "I'm usually careful and take my time, but I was angry and upset because it was so late and this lady had mentioned that she was not sure if she wanted the fur in the box after all. And so I just reached for the box, not taking my time to do it carefully," the client said.

The nursing measures were similar to the steps outlined for the previous client, with the addition of properly positioned pillows in bed to achieve a splinting effect. I explained about holding the body like a log whenever she turned, having preceded that action by lining up the body, contracting the abdominal and the gluteal muscles, and using the hands and arms and legs to push and to support the moving body. In two days, the client called me to thank me for the first nights of sleep she had had since the episode of hurting her back.

Client C

Another client in her late forties came to me because the medical care that had been prescribed had provided no relief. Several times she had been hospitalized for a number of days for innumerable tests to identify the cause of the back pain. All the test results had come back "negative." The doctors told her it was her nerves and prescribed a tranquilizer for her. The pain persisted. She told me, "I kept telling him that it is the muscles, but he said, 'No, I don't think so!' " The client had resorted to using an over-the-counter medication and heat, with the result that she had a small area of second-degree burns over her right lateral lumbar area. Her self-care assets were an awareness of the anatomy of the body and of the effectiveness of heat and massage for muscle ailments (although she used a cream with heat and that had caused the burns). Her self-care deficits were that she had not pursued to sufficient detail the physician's reasons for conducting the tests. My nursing measures were to encourage her to have confidence in her own judgments about her condition because she had made valids points in eliminating the likelihood of a ruptured intervertebral disc. "That would cause a pain that would follow the pathway of the nerve, wouldn't it?" she inquired. She also displayed reticence in asking a question about her approaching menopausal state. "Could the menopause be causing the pain in my back? You know, I feel I can ask you anything and talk about anything. The person who referred me to you said I should be sure to tell you everything, not to hold back anything that might be worrying me."

In the office, I checked the strength of the body of her muscles in her abdomen and in her back and found that there was strength in them; they had simply not been used. I demonstrated the posture that was prerequisite to the relief of the strain on the broad band of muscles bilaterally in the lumbar-sacral area and she gave evidence of understanding what the other measures were designed to achieve. As she was leaving the office she said, "You know, I feel better already."

Client example 24

One morning at 7:30 the phone rang in my apartment. The caller was a faculty member of a local university, a priest, who said there was a young lady with him in his office whom he thought I could help more than he could. I talked with the young lady, who was crying, and told her that I would be glad to see her right away in my office. We made an appointment for eight o'clock. When she entered my office, her eyes were very red from prolonged crying, her whole body was slumped into itself, her hair was limp, and it was obvious that she had not slept for a period of time. She had a haunted look about her and in her eyes there was a look that indicated a fear of herself, a fear that she lacked control over herself, a fear that something was wrong with her. As she began to speak, she talked in short, sometimes disconnected, sentences, would cry for a while, then resume, and gradually the sentences became more coherent as I gave her nursing care that would help her to pinpoint her need.

After several appointments, the following picture emerged. A male friend, with whom she had a platonic relationship, and with whom she shared responsibilities in a business venture, was constantly "dumping" on her, making her feel responsible for errors that had been made, making her feel as though her shortcomings were interfering with the happy re-lationship that had been enjoyed in the past. His gradually worsening attitude and silent treatment, as though he had been deeply hurt by her neglect, his shift in mood and behavior that was completely unpredictable, had made her feel totally inade-quate and had reduced her to an almost constant state of tears, loss of appetite, and finally, a fear that manifested itself in a physical reaction. When she heard his footsteps on the stairs, she would tremble as she waited for the knock on the door—actually a pounding on the door. She was eager to help him when he seemed to be discouraged and depressed. Sometimes he was sweet and appreciative of her friendship and concern; at other times he would belittle her with devastating remarks about her behavior or appearance in social situations or among friends. Several times, she had moved out of the situation, but always relented whenever he tracked her down and told her the business venture could not succeed without her and that he needed her. She would return to the close relationship necessi-tated by the demands of the business and the fact that they were both taking classes together. She wanted desperately to help him and felt that she was to blame for having difficulty in un-derstanding him. But his behavior had become so much more unpredictable that she now knew she had to get help to get out from under the depressing nature of the relationship. She was discerning that it was beginning to affect her ability to meet the requirements of courses, to accomplish everyday things in her own eyes; indeed, it was beginning to affect her total health state.

It took some time for her to develop insight into the situation because her insights into herself had been adulterated by vituperative, insinuating and accusatory vocal exchanges with the man, who actually had helped *her* in the past with difficult situations. She had had a high regard for him for a period of several years, and she had respected his opinions because he was highly intelligent, witty and clever. However, as she analyzed the situation, she was able to see those characteristics in a different light. "Now that I think about it. . . ," she would say, she could see that in many instances he had used his cleverness to manipulate people (carrying out deceptive actions with unmitigated boldness); to affront people; to confront people as if he himself had been the injured party when, for example, he tried to gain entrance to theaters or other buildings without tickets; and to execute paperwork involving legal angles. Gradually, the situation became clearer to my client, through the use of her self-care assets—the use of her power to reason, of her ability to look objectively and subjectively at herself, and to admit that the situation needed to be changed. She pondered the nursing measures that I prescribed: to focus on the undesirable aspects of the relationship whenever she felt herself "feeling sorry for him and wanting to help him"; to recognize that there was no evidence of improvement, but rather a deterioration of the relationship each time she resumed it after his insistence that he needed her. Eventually, she was able to accept the verbalization that his role in the relationship was essentially Svengalian, Rasputinian and most certainly malevolent in terms of the control that was being exercised over her. The client and I worked out a definitive method of terminating the relationship, with absolute secrecy about her plans and about where she would be living.

This summer, the client came to my office for an appointment to tell me how grateful she was for the help I had given her. She was beautiful in appearance now, virtually a different person, in control of herself, of her actions, of her life, and was continuing in school to prepare herself to be a lawyer.

It is interesting to note the circumstances prior to the phone call I received from the priest. When he arrived at the university that morning, the janitor and maid approached him and said, "Father, could you talk with this young lady? She has been here in the classroom since 6:30 this morning. She just keeps crying and saying she wants to talk to a priest; she has to talk to a priest." When Father took her into his office, she told him that once she had gone to a weekend encounter session conducted by a Catholic priest and that it had changed her whole life and her way of looking at things. Now that she needed help again, although she is not a Catholic, she turned immediately to a priest, and had come across town to a Catholic institution where she knew she could find one. Father had listened to her for a while, recognized that her problem was not a spiritual one, and that she was not in need of psychiatric help, since she was obviously making sense in her expression of her needs. Father said to me: "Where do other clergy send people like this, when they obviously need help from another professional, but do not need the kind of medical help that is available to them! She needed help right away. She needed you. She needed your nursing care. Thank God you were there and thank God I knew about you being there!"

Index